Skills of clinical supervision for nurses

SUPERVISION IN CONTEXT

Series editors:
Dr Peter Hawkins, Bath Consultancy Group
Robin Shohet, Centre for Staff Team Development, London and Scotland

---

Staff in all the helping professions are working under increasing amounts of pressure. They are having to balance growing levels of distress, disease and disturbance, while at the same time managing an increasing speed of change in the financing and organisational structures of their employing organisations. Staff will only stay effective at their important work if they are supported and well supervised. Often their supervisors move straight from being a skilled practitioner into a management and supervisory position, with no training in the skills that staff supervision requires.

This series is aimed at the increasing number of people who act as trainers, tutors, mentors and supervisors in the helping professions. It is also designed for those who are studying to become a trainer or supervisor and for supervisees, who can use the books to reflect on the many complex issues in their work.

The series is designed to follow on from the success of the bestselling title *Supervision in the Helping Professions* by Peter Hawkins and Robin Shohet. Each book explores the key issues, models and skills for trainers and supervisors in the main areas of the helping professions: social work and community care, the medical and nursing professions, psychotherapy, counselling and mentoring for managers.

Current titles:

Meg Bond and Stevie Holland: *Skills of Clinical Supervision for Nurses*
Allan Brown and Iain Bourne: *The Social Work Supervisor*

Skills of clinical supervision for nurses

A practical guide for supervisees, clinical supervisors and managers

**Meg Bond and
Stevie Holland**

Open University Press
Buckingham · Philadelphia

Open University Press
Celtic Court
22 Ballmoor
Buckingham
MK18 1XW

and
1900 Frost Road, Suite 101
Bristol, PA 19007, USA

First Published 1998

A catalogue record of this book is available from the British Library

ISBN 0 335 19660 8 (pb)   0 335 19661 6 (hb)

Library of Congress Cataloging-in-Publication Data
Bond, Meg.
    Skills of clinical supervision for nurses: a practical guide for
supervisees, clinical supervisors, and managers / Meg Bond and
Stevie Holland.
        p.   cm. — (Supervision in context)
    Includes bibliographical references and index.
    ISBN 0–335–19660–8 (pbk.). — ISBN 0–335–19661–8 (hbk)
    1. Nurses—Supervision of.   2. Nurses—Supervision of—Great
Britain.   I. Holland, Stevie, 1951– . II. Title. III. Series.
    [DNLM: 1. National Health Service (Great Britain) 2. Nursing,
Supervisory.   3. Nursing Care—organisation & administration.
4. Clinical Medicine—organisation & administration—nurses'
instruction.   5. Clinical Competence.   6. Mentors.   WY 105 B711s
1997]
RT86.45.B66   1997
362.1'73'0683—dc21
DNLM/DLC
for Library of Congress   97–15164
                                                                CIP

Typeset by Graphicraft Typesetters Ltd, Hong Kong
Printed in Great Britain by Biddles Ltd, Guildford and King's Lynn

Contents

Part I The context of clinical supervision in nursing

Part II Specific skills of clinical supervision

Part III   Organising clinical supervision systems

List of figures

List of tables

Series editors' preface

We welcome this book, the second in the series *Supervison in Context*, which looks at the particular supervision needs and issues in the various helping professions. The authors, Meg Bond and Stevie Holland, provide a timely contribution to the recent but growing literature on clinical supervison in nursing at a time when the rhetoric of clinical supervision is well ahead of the reality of practice in most organisations. To close the rift between the rhetoric and the reality requires much more emphasis on the understanding and training of effective nurse clinical supervisors, and this is the core focus of this book.

The first book in this series, *The Social Work Supervisor*, by Allan Brown and Iain Bourne, explored the many complex issues of supervising in the different settings where social work operates such as residential care, field social work, probation, hospitals and community development. Social work was the first of the helping professions to develop a strong culture of clinical supervision, not just for those who were in training but throughout the clinical career of the practitioner. Even in social work this culture has developed only over the last 20 years and is still far from established. In nursing the development of clinical supervision has started even more recently and the struggle to establish it as an essential aspect of clinical practice is far from complete. The authors welcome the policy initiatives on clinical supervision that have emanated from the UKCC and other bodies, while showing that practice lags behind. They argue that the need for effective clinical supervision is, in fact, becoming ever more urgent for the practitioner, the patient and the health of health organisations who are under ever-increasing pressures and demands. As they say in their Introduction:

> Clinical supervision provides a route to developing and maintaining emotionally healthier individuals in an emotionally healthier work-force culture. . . . Effective systems of clinical supervision can bring benefits not only to practitioners but also to the organisation and its clients.

This is particularly relevant now with the wave after wave of changes that are hitting the National Health Service. We believe that all change, however beneficial, involves some feelings of loss, and in the need to implement change, these feelings can get buried, with subsequent negative consequences. Clinical supervision can provide a safe forum for practitioners both to catch up with and work through their own reactions to these changes.

Meg Bond and Stevie Holland refer to the pioneering work of Isabel Menzies, who showed how the bureaucracy of the nursing practice and the many levels of nursing hierarchy served as a defence against the distress and anxiety that were a natural part of working with those who were disturbed, seriously ill or dying. In the nearly 40 years since Menzies carried out her study, there have been attempts to reduce the levels of hierarchy in nursing, to reduce the bureaucracy and to encourage nurses to develop closer relationships with their patients. However, if you reduce the institutional defence systems that provided emotional distance between nurse and patient, then it is essential to ensure that there are strong support systems for the nurse, who is more exposed to the emotional distress of the patient and their family.

When student nurses join the nursing profession we wonder how well they are informed about the likely effects on them of the emotional distress, dis-ease and disturbance of their patients. We suspect that it may still be seen as a weakness to be seen to be affected emotionally. However, we know, for example, that the grief of the family of a dying patient can restimulate past grief of the nurse, or a patient's fear can trigger different anxieties in the person working closely with them without that being in any way abnormal. In fact the non-recognition of how we are affected by others can itself become a problem, contributing to a culture of denial. We strongly support Meg Bond and Stevie Holland's case for clinical supervison as a way of breaking down such a culture.

As the institutional defences have been reduced there have been many initiatives in the nursing profession to develop support systems, such as mentoring, preceptorship, team work, peer support groups and clinical supervision. Meg Bond and Stevie Holland describe each of these processes and show the differing benefits of each system. Clearly their main focus is on clinical supervision and they forcibly argue for clinical supervision being separated out from managerial supervision wherever possible. This provides an equally important but contrasting viewpoint to our own book (Hawkins and Shohet 1989) and the first book in the series (Browne and Bourne 1996), which argue that managerial and clinical supervision can usefully be combined, and that there is much to be gained by focusing on the area of overlap between the two areas. Reactions to management changes in structures and systems, and feelings engendered by working with patients, can often cross-affect each other and take time to sort out. Meg Bond and Stevie Holland have the advantage of having spent many years as practitioners, supervisors and trainers in the nursing profession. From this position they passionately believe that managerial issues of assessment and control outweigh any possible benefits that might accrue from combining managerial and clinical supervision. However, even where the manager has little option but to provide the clinical supervision also, we believe there is much help and support they can receive from this book by learning how to separate the various aspects of their role and being sensitive to how their position of power affects the supervisee.

Having made a strongly argued case for regular clinical supervision for all nurses, Meg Bond and Stevie Holland show that establishing the supervision structure is not enough, for without trained and skilful supervisors effective supervision will not happen. The core of this book takes the reader through the key skills of effective clinical supervision and does so in a way that could be of great value not only to nurse supervisors but supervisors from all the other helping professions. They usefully adapt John Heron's model of six categories of possible interventions and show how they can be used, misused and abused in supervision. They also take the reader through steps to increase their own skills in each type of intervention.

Meg Bond and Stevie Holland are extremely well placed to write this book. They write, 'As nurses ourselves, we know well the foibles of our profession'. This leads them to ask (and answer in Chapter 2) such useful questions as why on earth has it taken so long to take clinical supervision on board, and why it might take longer still to implement effectively. In other words their enthusiasm and well-argued case do not gloss over potential difficulties.

As well as the experience of being practitioners themselves, they have both spent many years running training workshops for nurses and nurse supervisors. It is from these workshops and the questioning and needs of those attending that the models and approaches of this book have emerged:

> The strength of this book lies in the fact that it stems from contact with real practitioners, managers, professional support workers and educators in real settings . . . the frameworks . . . have sprung from our responses to the needs and concerns of people who attend our courses and who . . . want to make clinical supervision work.

We are sure that this excellent book will provide an invaluable contribution to the literature, and provide timely support to all those who 'want to make clinical supervision work'.

Acknowledgements

Our thanks to Robin for suggesting that we write the book and to Anna, Oriel, Elizabeth and Susan for special support. Many thanks to Shirley, Biddy and Rita (and her colleagues) for encouragement and advice. We much appreciated the tolerance of friends and family during our periods of isolation and irritability and especially Jo's vital sisterly humour and support (sorry the book isn't quite thick enough for you!). Special thanks to women's group members, Anna, Bette, Breda, Diana and Jill, for support and encouragement through post-bereavement writer's block and thanks also to Jacinta and Joan at Open University Press for kind understanding about the late delivery of the manuscript. Many thanks to Josie and Marie for such constructive and encouraging feedback on a draft of the manuscript. Special thanks to the people involved in our consultancy work and clinical supervision courses.

Introduction

This book is about the interpersonal and personal skills involved in clinical supervision in nursing, taking an approach which highlights focused growth and support as the vehicle for developing and sustaining quality clinical practice. We suggest that clinical supervision provides a route to developing and maintaining emotionally healthier individuals in an emotionally healthier workforce culture. We welcome the current impetus towards developing clinical supervision in nursing and echo Swain's sentiments that this may be overdue:

> It beggars belief that we have, for so long, failed to incorporate [clinical supervision] as a defined component of practice. Any one of us looking back at the human pain and social distress of others to which we have been exposed – not to mention our own – must surely question what makes us suppose we can practise effectively without such a regular conscientious examination of our work, of what might improve it, what might impede it, and of our own feelings about it.
>
> (Swain 1995: 12)

Effective systems of clinical supervision can bring benefits not only to practitioners but also to the organisation and its clients when it fulfils the aim of improving and developing clinical practice.

In our work as education and training consultants in the National Health Service, we find the most frequently asked questions about clinical supervision are 'What exactly IS it?' and 'How do we go about doing it?' From those who have begun to use clinical supervision, we are asked 'Are we doing it properly?' and those with more experience ask 'Why has it taken so long to get going in nursing?' Whilst participants on our skills training courses find some answers to these questions during the courses, many other practitioners have been frustrated with the lack of answers in the nursing literature. Our own search for practical guidance to help us with our confusion and uncertainty about clinical supervision in the nursing context has also been frustrating. Much work has had to be done by ourselves and our course participants to sift through and adapt theoretical models to make them practicable. This book attempts to share the results of this work by focusing on the *skills* of clinical supervision, thus giving a picture of what actually happens or could happen. Whilst no single page or chapter will adequately define clinical supervision or provide enough answers for everyone about how to do it well, the book as a whole will offer a sound practical basis for understanding, getting started and reviewing how you are progressing in using clinical supervision. Although our main focus is on practical frameworks which can help, we also want to be realistic and place them within the organisational context of what we know may be helpful or unhelpful to its development.

Clinical supervision is attracting a great deal of attention, energy and passion in the nursing literature and in practice areas. Experienced nurses who have survived many changes in nursing and management practice in recent years often view this enthusiasm with a certain amount of healthy cynicism: over-enthusiastic promotion of clinical supervision can make it sound like a holy grail. As with all holy grails, it attracts both devotees and non-believers and it is the search that can often attract the most attention and noise. Many pilgrims flock to support it, some out of genuine belief, some because it's the fashionable thing to do. Many may pay lip service to the creed but, either wittingly or unwittingly, will be highly selective or shallow in putting it into everyday practice. Many will view it simply as the unearthing of old relics and scriptures which they had problems worshipping the first time around. Many more will be indifferent to the entire pilgrimage, preferring to conduct their working lives without recall to any other image.

Whilst we too feel enthusiastic about clinical supervision, we would like this book to be a realistic, practical guide, rather than a heroic crusade. We include the reality of the difficulties that you may encounter in developing clinical supervision, signposting some of those challenges that cannot be spirited away. As nurses ourselves, we know well the foibles of our profession, such as the tendency to strive for perfection, with the inevitable discouragement that ensues from not achieving it. Other professions which have implemented clinical supervision decades ago have not achieved perfection and neither will we. The 'good enough' clinical supervision referred to by Hawkins and Shohet (1989) requires a balanced view, both of the very real potential benefits of clinical supervision and an exploration of some of the limitations and barriers it might face. Some of these barriers come from within ourselves as individual nurses and from within the culture of our profession. As authors we might be interpreted as being critical in challenging these. However, our deep concern is to ensure that clinical supervision works well enough in nursing to provide the support and growth opportunities that nurses deserve in doing a difficult job in a difficult political and organisational climate. Our patients and clients deserve to be cared for by people with the backup of 'good enough' clinical supervision.

Who this book is for

This book is aimed at every nurse, midwife and health visitor and their managers, professional support workers and educators who have an interest in the practical implementation of clinical supervision. This is potentially a vast number of people within a huge diversity of contexts and experience. We are conscious of the fact that nursing encompasses a very wide range of settings and that nurses can be insular within their own discipline. The book focuses on the principles and skills of developmental clinical supervision that can be applied, sometimes with local adaptation, across the board. The examples given will illustrate the type of issues that frequently emerge in our workshops. However, we accept that we cannot describe specific application of the principles of clinical supervision to every setting in nursing, midwifery and health visiting and we trust that you will be able to use your imagination to relate what we offer in this book to your own speciality.

Note: the midwifery profession has developed a specific system of clinical supervision that differs from many of the principles we put forward in this book. However, midwives who wish to extend and deepen their use of their clinical supervision system will also find the emphasis on skills in this book useful.

Terms used

Usually when one wishes to be inclusive of all branches of the profession, one uses the full title of 'nursing, midwifery and health visiting'. In the attempt to be succinct, we will use 'nursing' as shorthand, meaning to include all nurses as well as health visitors, midwives, managers, professional support workers and educators. The term 'practitioners' is used to include all nurses, midwives and health visitors who work directly with patients or clients. We use the term 'clients' as a generic term to include patients, clients, relatives, carers and any client groups.

If we cannot find a non-clumsy, non-gender-specific way of referring to people of both sexes, both practitioner and client will be referred to as 'she' (which reflects the statistical preponderance of women in both these groups).

How to use this book

The breadth and depth of the human skills involved in clinical supervision are potentially vast and it is only humanly possible to explore one or two aspects at a time. Therefore each chapter in this book is designed to enable you to explore a very limited part of the overall picture. The analogy of gymnasium exercises could be useful here. In the gym, you focus on specific groups of muscles and ligaments at a time to stretch and strengthen them, so that back in the world outside the gym, you have more physical strength, flexibility, coordination and self-awareness of your physical abilities and limitations. Likewise in the skills approach in this book, we focus on specific aspects to help you to stretch and strengthen your awareness and understanding of the specific skills of clinical supervision and to recognise your strengths and weaknesses. As a result, we hope that you will be able to apply your learning to the real-life clinical supervision situation with greater skill, flexibility, confidence in your abilities and knowledge of your limitations.

We are alert to the points highlighted in Alison Norman's summing up of a National Health Service Management Executive's (NHSME) workshop on clinical supervision, in which she said that a one-dimensional, inflexible approach to clinical supervision would be a tragedy for nursing: 'we have a history in our professions of having very good ideas and trying to put them in tablets of stone, when they should be fluid and instilled within each individual organisation' (Norman 1995: 24). There are more specific guidelines in this book than is usual in the literature so far, where writers are cautious about being over-prescriptive about such a variable interpersonal process. However, in offering our ideas, practical guidelines, structures and ways of identifying skills, we encourage you to use them selectively and to adapt them to your own situation. We do not see them as definitive: there are no tablets of stone.

We have attempted to apply the discipline of describing each of these as 'a framework for . . .' rather than 'a model'. The use of the term 'model' implies a replica, giving a fairly detailed impression of the shape and colour of the finished product, perhaps like an architect's model of a proposed building. We prefer the term 'framework' since we offer our ideas as mere frames upon which to hang your work: more like a weaver's loom, with no expectation of the colours and textures that you will create; we merely hope to make it easier for you to weave your own pattern. We have great concern about the proliferation and interpretation of 'models' of clinical supervision in nursing. We find on the one hand that nurses with an academic background can tend to collect 'models' of clinical supervision without getting round to erecting the building. Some discussions on courses can degenerate into a 'who can quote the most models?' competition, with avoidance of taking the first step of putting anything into practice. Some other nurses, desperate to get started with clinical supervision in this time of great need, adopt one model and try to apply it universally to everyone and every issue ('we are using So-and-So's model of clinical supervision'). We hope that this book will enable you to say 'we are doing clinical supervision our way' rather than paying us the dubious and unwelcome compliment of 'we are using Bond and Holland's model of clinical supervision'. So, we expect you to select and adapt any of the ideas and structures which illuminate, help you to understand, enable you to put into practice some aspect of clinical supervision or review your use of it more effectively. We hope that you will ignore those that are not useful to you now, and that perhaps you will revisit them another time if appropriate.

Contents of the book

Part I, 'The Context of Clinical Supervision in Nursing', sets the scene for understanding the special context of clinical supervision in nursing, the organisational impetus for the development of clinical supervision and the factors which have blocked its progress so far, and may continue to do so if not attended to. There are two chapters in Part I, which, although they interlock, explore similar themes from different perspectives.

Chapter 1 gives the surface picture of clinical supervision, outlines its key principles, its roots in other professions, their influences, the early developments and writings related specifically to nursing and the ideological and organisational factors which are a spur to the development of clinical supervision. In short, the good news. We look at why the need to implement clinical supervision has become so important in nursing. We need to place it in context – why clinical supervision, why now at this stage in nursing history, what is its purpose and value? We wish to place clinical supervision in the current organisational, educational and clinical milieux as we see them.

Chapter 2 introduces you to the more 'hidden' picture – the pitfalls, resistances and difficulties the development of clinical supervision is likely to meet on the way, both from individuals and from the prevailing culture of the health service itself: the bad news. We address the questions: why on earth has it taken so long and why might it take longer still, to implement effectively? We explore how and why some of its principles may be less well received than others in the current climate and within the complex folds of our huge profession. We view these blocks as being a matter of individual and organisational psychology.

Our intention is to place the emotional life of clients, practitioners, supervisors, managers and the larger organisation firmly in the centre of this book and this chapter sets the scene for this. We don't intend that you should become a 'barefoot therapist', but wish to avoid a shallow 'soundbite approach' to clinical supervision which pretends it can be implemented by knitting on additional practical strategies without reference to what really makes people (and organisations) tick. This superficial approach would result in your emotional feelings about your clients, your colleagues, yourself, and about how you practise staying 'out of mind' whilst retaining their power. Chapter 2 explores how practitioners in health care have cultivated their defences against recognising the emotional underpinning of many of their interactions with others. It also seeks to identify how unconscious emotional responses are mirrored and transmitted between all participants in health care and outlines the impact and influence this can have on the relationship in clinical supervision. Everyone who has some role in implementing clinical supervision needs to understand how unconscious forces can impact in different ways on the entire process. The pitfalls identified in the skills chapters in Part II are linked to these hidden restraints.

Part II, 'Specific Skills of Clinical Supervision', is the largest and most important part of the book as it is concerned with clarifying and encouraging development of specific skills of clinical supervision and highlighting the possible pitfalls. We begin in Chapter 3 to set the scene for the clinical supervision relationship and offer some frameworks for building and sustaining a working alliance. We suggest some ways of structuring the clinical supervision relationship to enhance its quality and prevent and deal with some of the hidden problems which can emerge to sabotage the process. We are aware that this interpersonal dimension is a vast arena and have there-fore selected frameworks that have proved to be in most demand and of most use to our course participants: clarifying the rights and responsibilities of supervisee and clinical supervisor, negotiating a working contract, review-ing the progress of the working alliance and dealing with criticism.

Chapters 4, 5 and 6 examine the specific skills required to do the work that the clinical supervision relationship is set up to achieve. The skills of the supervisee in preparing for and using the time for in-depth reflection on practice are examined in Chapter 4, which takes a practical approach by offering some frameworks for thinking that have helped nurses get started and review their progress. It does not claim to be an exhaustive account of the vast literature on reflective practice in nursing: this has more usefully been done elsewhere (Palmer *et al.* 1994).

Chapter 5 emphasises the importance of the non-directive skills of support and catalytic facilitation which are the basis of the help that the clinical supervisor can give the supervisee. While there are commonalities with use of counselling skills, we try to put these in the context of clinical supervision rather than counselling sessions, with some possible pitfalls signposted.

Chapter 6 attempts to clarify the importance of the authoritative (not authoritarian) or directive aspects of clinical supervision. Skills of challeng-ing the supervisee are placed alongside the skills of offering support towards change; and the skills of giving information and advice are set alongside catalytic skills of enabling the supervisee to use the information to make their own informed decisions.

Chapters 3, 4, 5 and 6 tend to focus on and illustrate the one-to-one clin-ical supervision scenario, while Chapter 7 extends the frameworks offered in these early chapters to the group clinical supervision context. Additional frameworks for understanding the skills involved in group clinical supervi-sion are offered, along with some structures to enhance the quality of the group work and prevent and deal with some of the additional hidden prob-lems which can emerge to sabotage the process of a group. The aim is to ensure that effective clinical supervision can occur in the relationship dynamic of the group setting.

Part III, 'Organising Clinical Supervision Systems', of the book is a one-chapter section, providing guidelines for managers and coordinators to set up, monitor and develop clinical supervision delivery frameworks. We dis-tinguish between clinical supervision and management supervision, by iden-tifying some of the elements of the interaction and how they differ between the two types of supervision. We do not wish to suggest that management supervision is bad and clinical supervision is good; just that this book focuses on the skills of clinical supervision not management supervision, and that guidance about the skills of the latter (valid, important and necessary) rela-tionship should be sought elsewhere.

It suggests some conditions which are necessary for the development of effective clinical supervision relationships into working alliances and some options from which to choose an appropriate delivery framework for clinical supervision in your organisation. A framework is offered to guide you through the steps involved in setting up a clinical supervision system and some pitfalls are highlighted. Suggestions are made for methods to monitor and evaluate clinical supervision, within the limitations of the difficulties of finding relevant evaluation tools for assessing such a relationship-based system which is notoriously difficult to measure. We also point to possible developments in clinical supervision in the future and highlight some issues that need to be addressed for the future success of clinical supervision in nursing.

Your starting point in reading this book will depend on your learning style. On our courses we find that some people need to have a rationale and context-setting introduction before trying out the skills building exercises, while others learn better by getting on with the practical side and addressing the questions that arise as they go along. Likewise, some may prefer to begin reading this book at Part I and then look at the more practical sections. Others will prefer to go straight to Parts II or III and then flip back to Part I when they begin to wonder why we use a particular approach. Of course, the choice is yours.

Background to the book

The strength of this book lies in the fact that it stems from contact with real practitioners, managers, professional support workers and educators in real settings. Our interactive, experiential workshops and consultancy work in various NHS Trusts attempt to mirror the interpersonal principles espoused in this book. Thus the frameworks on offer here have sprung from our responses to the needs and concerns of people who attend our courses and who (mostly) want to make clinical supervision work. The relationships we have made with these people have included brave disclosures of their own feelings, thoughts and experiences. We have studied the theoretical background to clinical supervision in nursing and we were involved with some early attempts to develop clinical supervision when we were working in clinical nursing practice. However, we have learned immeasurably more about the realities of clinical supervision in practice, and about its true potential, from the truths that these people have shared about their working lives and the part they play as human beings in their work. We would like to thank them for working so generously with us.

In an attempt not to abuse the trust and openness of these people, confidentiality has been maintained in the use of real-life examples and quotations in this book (all the case examples and quotations come from our workshops and consultancy work). We have changed names, settings and often amalgamated other details so that individual patient, nurse and organisational confidentiality are not compromised. All the examples or quotations were witnessed or heard within the confidentiality contracts of skills training courses or consultancy within Trusts; we are therefore not at liberty to reveal sources.

We could not have written this without our own unique experiences of receiving clinical supervision to ground the theory and ideas into our own inner as well as external reality. We have both received clinical supervision for many years and are grateful to the supervisors and groups involved. We also provide clinical supervision for others working in our field and have learned much from these working alliances.

Part I
The context of clinical supervision in nursing

1 ▷ The surface picture: the development and value of clinical supervision

This chapter gives a brief overview of the context of clinical supervision in nursing today. We focus on the sources and development of ideas within it and the perceived value of implementing clinical supervision for both individual practitioners and the organisation as a whole. Fuller accounts of the principles, aims, models of clinical supervision are given elsewhere (Butterworth and Faugier 1992; Kohner 1994; Fowler 1996). Our aim is to highlight aspects of this development which we believe will ensure fundamental and effective change and a healthier work environment.

What exactly is clinical supervision?

Since clinical supervision is a relationship between human beings, it is difficult to pinpoint exactly in one succinct definition what it is about. The variety of helping relationships have much in common, from work-based relationships such as practitioner/client and support between colleagues, to personal relationships such as friendships and family interactions. They all aim towards meeting basic human needs, and when reduced to their basic components, look very much alike.

There are as many written definitions of clinical supervision as there are published books and papers on the subject: each author highlights the elements which are most important to them. Before we add our own definition, we would like to highlight some of the loaded meanings that the term clinical supervision seems to have for nurses. These loaded meanings come to the fore fairly soon in any discussion between nurses about clinical supervision and we feel it is important to acknowledge them before presenting an ideal alternative.

First, 'clinical' may be an uncomfortable prefix for many practitioners engaged in health care, who may believe it to be too embedded in a medical model approach. Minimalist interpretations of 'clinical' may ensure that only the 'what' and 'how' of immediate technical aspects of care are emphasised;

it could be used principally in a reactive way to maintain baseline standards. For some the term 'clinical' obscures a more critical overview of the broader complexities and context of practice, as well as the wider and more important remit of personal and professional development.

Second, the term 'supervision' may also be met with suspicion. Its general meaning is concerned with 'keeping an eye on someone', checking that work is being done appropriately and effectively and, as such, its more context-specific application in nursing can result in its being tainted with a negative image. For some, it automatically smacks of being looked at critically through a magnifying glass, a one-way process of observation and control. In an early example of the clinical supervision process in health visiting, the health visitors and their manager in Stepney were clearly antagonistic to the term 'supervision' for these reasons (Kohner 1994). Such negative views perhaps reflect the very real experiences of many practitioners who have worked in a predominantly non-supportive and hyper-critical climate (Bond 1986; Woodhouse and Pengelly 1991). Although on a rational level many practitioners may realise that clinical supervision is supposed to be a helpful and supportive process, it is important to acknowledge that more jaundiced and confused perceptions exist and these may distort initial understanding and assimilation of the ideas related to it.

So, many begin their exploration of clinical supervision confused about its meaning and about how it compares to and differs from other support initiatives such as preceptorship, mentoring, supervised practice or peer support. This is not surprising. Clinical supervision is in its infancy period in nursing, and yet it is being forced to face the dilemma of having to grow up very fast. Due to the nature and speed of change within the NHS and our profession, there are many pressures to implement it quickly. Despite the absence of clinical data about implementation and effectiveness, criticised and mourned by Fowler (1996), many are exploring how it can be translated and applied within our vast and diverse profession. The task ahead is a large and daunting one and many are rushing ahead without first really examining the ideas within clinical supervision and their attitudes to it, to see which feel most appropriate and applicable to their speciality or location.

We offer our own, inevitably incomplete, attempt at definition, though we emphasise that it cannot stand alone without an examination of the principles behind it:

> Clinical supervision is regular, protected time for facilitated, in-depth reflection on clinical practice. It aims to enable the supervisee to achieve, sustain and creatively develop a high quality of practice through the means of focused support and development. The supervisee reflects on the part she plays as an individual in the complexities of the events and the quality of her practice. This reflection is facilitated by one or more experienced colleagues who have expertise in facilitation and the frequent, ongoing sessions are led by the supervisee's agenda. The process of clinical supervision should continue throughout the person's career, whether they remain in clinical practice or move into management, research or education.

We would like to expand on this definition by addressing some simple yet contentious questions.

- What are the key principles that underpin clinical supervision?
- who should offer clinical supervision?
- who should receive clinical supervision?
- how does it relate to other support mechanisms endorsed within the organisation of nursing?

Principles of clinical supervision

We would like to begin by identifying some key characteristics of clinical supervision. We will be highlighting those characteristics which are most congruent with our own values as outlined in the Introduction and which will be fleshed out later in the 'practical' part of the book. We refer to the writers whose work has most engaged our attention and that of the practitioners with which we have worked. We also highlight some of the ambivalence as to how these principles may be put into practice.

For many, the importance of clinical supervision is that it focuses its lens clearly on clinical practice – how practitioners engage with clients for the benefits of clients, to improve care and standards and to develop personal/ professional skills and satisfaction. Butterworth (1995: 4) states that his preference is for a definition which encapsulates the 'heart' of clinical supervision – 'that which talks clearly about sustaining and developing nursing' – and that the focus for this should clearly be the clinician actively engaged in clinical practice. '[Clinical supervision is] . . . an exchange between practising professionals to enable the development of professional skills . . . We must jealously guard our excellence and skills in clinical practice, and sustain and develop them' (Butterworth 1995: 12). By placing a microscope on clinical practice he goes on to suggest that clinical supervision offers protection to independent and accountable practice, but only if it is built into professional life – 'it requires time and energy and is not just an incidental event' (1995: 4).

It is clear that if the importance of clinical practice needs to be restored, then it requires personal commitment from individuals as well as commitment from the organisation to ensure its effectiveness and enshrine it within the structure of professional life. Swain (1995: 19) asserts that 'the prime aim [of clinical supervision] is to restore the centrality of professional clinical practice to the health service'. She suggests that for too long the shifting political games have blurred and distorted the picture of service provision away from this central purpose. The 'lens' of clinical supervision may be used to magnify specific features of clinical practice or to make a wide-angled sweep of the context of practice.

This lens analogy can be carried to another concept nurses find helpful. Houston's (1990) simple suggestion of highlighting the SUPER in clinical supervision serves to emphasise the far-seeing element and unhook it from more negative emotional loading alluded to earlier. SUPERvision helps to shift the perspective from more 'myopic' vision, focusing only on what we can spot right in front of our eyes, which tends to become concentrated into what has not been achieved, or on errors in judgement or practice. A broader view then allows for an overview of past, present and future professional work, as well as an in-depth exploration of specific interventions and feelings and reactions in particular situations.

The interpersonal qualities needed within the clinical supervision relationship should be highlighted, to ensure that it is both effective and humane. Faugier (1992: 24) endorses and writes sensitively about, the need for a 'growth and support' model: 'The role of the supervisor is to facilitate *growth* both educationally and personally in the supervisee, whilst providing essential *support* to their developing clinical autonomy'. She goes on to suggest qualities needed in the clinical supervision relationship to enable this, namely: generosity, openness, willingness to learn, encouragement, intellectual stimulation, humanity, sensitivity and uncompromising rigour. Swain (1995) is particularly eloquent about the need for nurses to develop a more nurturing and truly supportive climate for each other, one that might be more compatible with the aims of their role:

> Something more is clearly needed to help practitioners . . . attention to the needs of staff themselves: to their workloads, their professional practice and concerns and anxieties about it: to their feeling state and health state; to their capacity for creative work, and its encouragement, and to establishing a place of safety where disappointment or failure in practice can be examined honestly; prejudices challenged constructively, and success and good work owned and applauded.
>
> (1995: 19)

As Faugier (1992) suggests, clinical supervision should be about empowerment and not control, hence emphasising that the route to professional accountability is through building confidence and self-esteem, which in turn requires careful, supportive feedback. Swain's view seeks to challenge the lack of congruence between the caring vocabulary used by practitioners in their treatment of clients and the distinctly unsupportive if not harsh attitudes and actions reserved for each other. This has been compounded in certain policy directives which have contained punitive statements concerning practitioners taking sick leave. Reluctance to 'admit' stress is endemic at all levels in the NHS. It may be argued that there is often a huge gap between the concept of empowerment and its true espousal and implementation. Clinical supervision may offer a practical mechanism and forum in which to practise and develop these skills and enable the growth of clinical leadership, which has suffered such erosion in recent years (Rafferty 1993).

The capacity for, and skills in, reflective practice are key components of clinical supervision and contribute to its essential educational function. For over ten years reflective practice has been given much value in the nursing literature, emphasising the need to build space to implement reflective processes in nursing. However, the reality is that there has been a marked lack of time or will for this to happen in practice. Our experience and that of many qualified practitioners with which we work suggests that instances of good reflective practice are much more scarce than the literature might suggest. Clinical supervision potentially provides the medium in which to structure space and time for reflection although it still needs the personal and organisational commitment to protect it from the erosion of other competing organisational commitments. Critical reflection enables a balance and an alliance between feelings, intuition, emotional skills, cognitive insights and theoretical links. It has a capacity to inform and assist both personal and professional development.

Many have referred to the all-important need for both players in the clinical supervision relationship to develop skills in self-awareness. Woods (1992) emphasises the emotional underpinning of clinical supervision and therapeutic use of self within the clinical supervision relationship. He also rightly examines the organisational and cultural context in which this takes place and the limited extent to which permission is given to both acknowledge and develop emotional skills. Platt-Koch (1986) tries to balance the educational function of clinical supervision with the therapeutic nature of the relationship: 'In supervision, the nurse gains theoretical knowledge but also learns to make new and fuller use of self'. However, there is some ambivalence as to how this might be achieved and sometimes a sense of embarrassment about endorsing it completely. For example, Faugier (1992: 19) highlights the therapeutic origins of clinical supervision and the therapeutic intention and outcomes implicit in her 'growth and support' model, but she then seems to water the message down: 'The real purpose of supervision . . . is the promoting of learning about nursing, including some personal growth content'. She then suggests that it is neither possible nor desirable for all nurses to shift their philosophical orientation from nursing to psychotherapeutic, social or educational models. We would suggest that these are all part of the clinical supervision relationship and all part of nursing. However, it is very important that attention is paid to boundaries for and skills in their application.

There seems to be the viewpoint that if too much attention is given to these subterranean emotions, they might undermine the educative function of clinical supervision completely. That confusing mixed messages exist here is not surprising. Despite nurses, midwives and health visitors working in the highly emotional and vulnerable arena of health and ill-health, where the fear or reality of illness and disability can challenge personal autonomy and the very sense of who we are, there can be a deep reluctance to give space for emotional expression. The extent to which clinical supervision can provide this opportunity remains highly contentious. We will explore the reasons for this deep ambivalence and resistance as well as the real difficulties in achieving appropriate balance between personal and professional components of clinical supervision in Chapter 2.

Some authors suggest a combination of principal purposes which try to bring together and provide a more composite picture of the personal and professional developmental model of clinical supervision. For Platt-Koch (1986), the aims of supervision are to expand knowledge base, develop clinical expertise and proficiency, and develop self-esteem and autonomy.

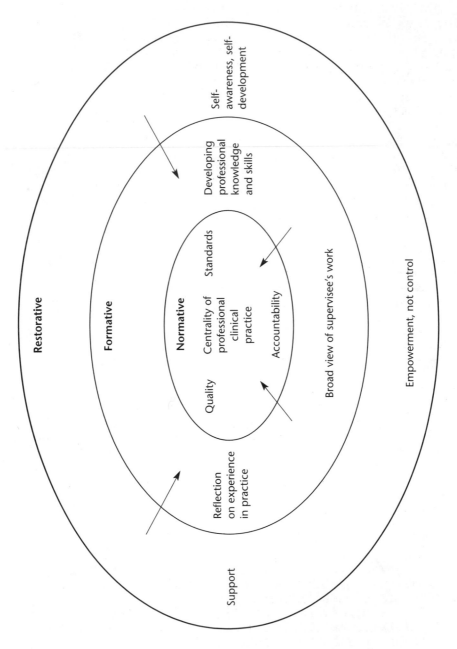

Figure 1.1 The restorative and formative functions of clinical supervision are the means by which the normative function is addressed

The Department of Health (1993d: 15) defines clinical supervision as:

the term used to describe a formal process of professional support and learning which enables practitioners to develop knowledge and competence, assume responsibility for their own practice and enhance consumer protection and the safety of care in complex clinical situations. It is central to the process of learning and to the expansion of the scope of practice and should be seen as the means for encouraging self assessment and analytic and reflective skills . . .

To this we would add emotional skills. One of the most widely quoted integrated descriptions is Proctor's (1986) trio of formative, normative and restorative functions. The formative function of supervision is about developing the skills, understanding and abilities of the supervisee through an in-depth reflection of the supervisee's work with clients. The normative function highlights the importance of professional and organisational standards and the need for competence and accountability, whilst with the 'restorative function' Proctor (1986: 24) clearly acknowledges the supportive remit of supervision:

[it is] a way of supporting workers who are affected by the distress, pain and fragmentation of the client and how they need time to become aware how this has affected them and to deal with reactions. This is essential if workers are not to become over full of emotions, or alternatively heavily defended against the distress of the client, therefore lacking empathy and good-enough care.

We adapt Proctor's (1986) framework in Figure 1.1, which emphasises that the means by which the normative function is addressed is through the medium of the restorative and formative functions. This diagram incorporates the principles we have outlined so far in this chapter.

We will be exploring the main influences on the development of clinical supervision in the last part of this chapter – the 'push factors' that have ensured their frequent, if erratic, appearance in the literature. Chapter 2 will outline the 'blocking' factors that get in the way of effective application of these principles. The rest of the book will focus on the skills necessary to actualise them.

These principles provide practitioners in diverse health care situations with a flexible framework of clinical supervision that can benefit the practitioner, their practice and ultimately the client. They may explore and harness each principle to an appropriate degree, achieving the balance needed to meet very different situations and requirements. There may be a very different balance required by practitioners in accident and emergency who have come through a major critical incident, compared to community paediatric nurses supporting families with chronically sick children at home. Clearly the balance may be affected by the location and nature of service provision – from acute high tech, public health, acute low tech, community practice, cottage hospital, general practitioner's surgery, learning disability teams, hospital and community midwives, secure units and so on – and, by the degree of practitioner experience and stage of their career, as well as by the myriad different personal histories and needs of staff in these diverse fields of practice.

All these underpinning principles need to be acknowledged and worked with in the clinical supervision relationship although some principles may predominate at some times more than others. What we are suggesting is that acute imbalances make for a very different total experience of clinical supervision and the person selected (or volunteering) for the role of clinical supervisor may serve to shift the balance of this entire framework. If the person in the role of clinical supervisor is also a manager then the normative elements could easily attain prominence, whilst the supervisee's (and indeed the manager/supervisor's) vulnerabilities, stresses and support needs may disappear or go into hiding. This is why we are strongly recommending that managers do not assume a clinical supervisor role with any of their own staff. This theme will reappear throughout the book.

Who should be clinical supervisors?

Qualified senior staff, with more than or equal experience to that of the intended supervisees should be selected. Although managers may play a role in identifying appropriate clinical supervisors, there should not be any enforced conscription for this role as it involves a great deal of commitment. They should usually (although not always) be from the same clinical area or with sufficient recent experience of relevant clinical practice. These clinical supervisors need to undergo further skills training to equip them for this role. (These skills will be explored fully in Parts II and III.) It needs to be said that seniority does not always denote appropriate levels of experience. Sadly, expertise is not a quality automatically distilled from years of service. We can all think of people who would consider themselves to be wise elders, and yet whose attitudes are stuck in a bygone age and who seem to have learned little from the intervening years.

We are clearly emphasising the need for clinicians in the role of clinical supervisor and strongly endorse the inappropriateness of having line managers in this role. 'Management supervision and clinical supervision are different functions and should not be undertaken by the same person', Margaret Buttegieg declares (in the introduction to Swain 1995: 5) in a clear message on behalf of the CPHVA. This has been echoed by many from other nursing specialities in both acute and community settings and has been endorsed by the UKCC (1996). Senior managers have an extremely important role in facilitating the development of supervision systems in identifying and providing resources for training, in its evaluation and in making a case for its inclusion within service contracts (see Part III). But any embodiment of clinical supervision within management will be liable to cause confusion and mistrust and lead to mixed messages about its aims and potential.

Management-led clinical supervision could lead to restrictive practice rather than reflective and growthful practice. We realise that some practitioners and managers may disagree with this, although all practitioners on our workshops have supported this view and most managers who have participated have returned to base to rethink their intended implementation locally. This is supported by Swain's (1995) own experience in workshop feedback. In specific areas of practice, notably throughout midwifery and in some instances of child protection, a form of management-led clinical supervision is already in progress. We know that many in reality will also follow this approach. We hope that even if your views differ you will find ample ideas in this book to aid your role and allow the developmental rather than punitive aspects to flourish. Specific guidance for managers on how to use this book is given in Chapter 8.

Who should receive clinical supervision?

We believe that all qualified practitioners in all clinical areas need clinical supervision to maintain proficiency in practice, to ensure their accountability and to aid their specific personal and professional growth and development. This includes those who have had additional training to become clinical supervisors. We believe that no one has achieved such a hallowed status that they are above needing clinical supervision. We also believe that all related personnel – teachers and managers – should also be in receipt of clinical supervision. This acknowledges the challenge made to all professionals, that their initial qualification is only a passport to practice and that it is necessary to endorse mechanisms which ensure continued professional competence (Jarvis 1983).

Clinical supervision can contribute to this lifelong need to update, improve and develop and does so by being firmly rooted in the work context. Few are 'qualified enough' or expert enough never to need help and guidance with their own developmental process at some time. We are aware that in such a large profession as ours, the means for achieving such extensive clinical supervision networks will need carefully planned and layered training programmes and will take a lot of time, effort and resources. However, its universality is crucial.

Not until recently has clinical supervision been seen as the right and responsibility of every practitioner. However, many may still find it more comforting to regard it as appropriate only for those who are in difficulty, those who are not maintaining standards or those who are encountering particularly stressful, acute or complex situations. This emphasis on 'problem' versus growth and development in nursing can be difficult to let go of, just as the espousal of illness rather than health has been for many within the NHS.

Comparisons with other structured organisational support mechanisms

The principles of personal and professional support and guidance have been more easily endorsed for new practitioners and for those returning to practice after a break. This is possibly why clinical supervision is frequently

Table 1.1   Distinguishing between some structured support systems in nursing

	Mentorship	Preceptorship	Supervised practice	Peer support	Clinical supervision
Supervisee	Student nurse	Newly qualified nurse or qualified nurse entering a new field	Student health visitor on final fieldwork placement	Any nurse	Qualified nurse
Period of time	Throughout training especially on practical placements	During the 6 to 12 months of adjustment	The final three months of the HV course	Varies; support groups have a reputation for petering out	Intended to be throughout career
How widespread	Integral part of the course	Varies; likely to become more widespread	Integral part of the course	Patchy; not widely accepted	Patchy, rapidly accelerating
Assessment function	Mentor often has a part to play in assessment of practical work	Preceptor may report to supervisee's manager	Supervisor has a defined assessment role: HV cannot qualify without passing this part of the course	No assessment function, colleagues do not report to anyone unless there is evidence of unsafe or unethical practice	No assessment function, clinical supervisor does not report to anyone unless there is evidence of unsafe or unethical practice

confused with preceptorship and mentoring schemes. There is an added history here of blurring of terminology and confusion in the teaching/assessing and general supportive aspects of these roles. How is clinical supervision similar to and how is it different from these and other more informal support schemes? (See Table 1.1.)

Preceptor support

Preceptorship is aimed at facilitating the sometimes stressful transition from student to newly qualified practitioner and helping build confidence in that new role. The preceptor has an educative and modelling function, enabling the new practitioner to develop new skills and aiding the application of theory to practice; and ideally 'allows for a smooth transition from learner to accountable practitioner' (Morton-Cooper and Palmer 1993: 99). The difficulties of applying what was originally a US-grown model of preceptorship, which was akin to an apprenticeship learning system, to different educational and service models in the UK has been well documented (Butterworth 1992; Morton-Cooper and Palmer 1993).

The UKCC's (1993) guidance on preceptor support differs in that it emphasises that it is a relationship between two qualified practitioners, both of whom are accountable for their practice. The more experienced participant works in partnership to guide the newly qualified practitioner in adapting to their new role. The preceptor needs to have had at least 12 months' or equivalent experience within the same clinical field. The guidance stresses the support required from the preceptor to assist in the 'beginner's' adjustment to new responsibilities.

The earlier work of Kramer (1974) had outlined the danger zone time of transition as one which could create the stressful burden of 'reality shock'. Ironically, as our own work with returners to practice suggests, part of that reality shock may involve dealing with the intransigence and poor role modelling of those in a preceptor role (Holland 1994). The difference between the intended remit of the preceptor role and the reality of the joint experience depends upon the quality of preceptor selection and the training available. Morton-Cooper and Palmer (1993) refer to the resource difficulties in obtaining enough willing practitioners for this role and the likely problems of coercion in what should be a creative and sensitive learning relationship. Words of warning indeed for those setting up clinical supervision systems or those being persuaded to become clinical supervisors before they are ready.

It is interesting to note that some of the early references to supervision in health visiting (Fish *et al* 1989) seem to refer to the period of supervised practice towards the end of this post-registration course. These are more reminiscent of the need to guide and support the newly qualified practitioner than clinical supervision per se.

Mentor support

Mentor schemes have gathered momentum in the last decade in the UK and have gained increasing prominence particularly within nurse education programmes, specifically within Project 2000, to assist with educational input and support in the practice setting. Much of the research stems from America, with, as Butterworth (1992) suggests, dubious applicability to nursing in the UK. The role of mentors has been subject to much debate. Some suggest that they possess very similar characteristics to preceptors; the two terms have been known to be used interchangeably. Morton-Cooper and Palmer (1993) allude to the confusion in terminology now being added to by the additional concept of clinical supervision. Mentoring involves experienced practitioners who nurture and guide students in clinical placements but also have an active educational element. There is some contention whether they also have a role in assessment. It is based on a one-to-one method of teaching and facilitation, the content and direction of which should be negotiated by both parties in joint planning.

Others would suggest that assessment was not compatible with the supportive functions of the mentor.

> Mentoring concerns the building of a dynamic relationship in which the personal characteristics, philosophies and priorities of the individual members interact to influence in turn the nature, direction and duration of the resulting, eventual partnership. What lies at the heart of the process is the shared, encouraging and supportive elements that are based on mutual attraction and common values. These . . . facilitate the personal development and career/professional socialisation for the mentoree – leading to eventual reciprocal benefits for both parties. A mentoring relationship is one that is enabling and cultivating; a relationship that assists in empowering an individual within the working environment.
>
> (Morton-Cooper and Palmer 1993: 59)

They advocate that the person with the role of mentor needs a repertoire of helper functions – adviser, coach, counsellor, sponsor, teacher, resource facilitator – a menu to be mixed and matched. Morton-Cooper and Palmer's (1993) buoyantly enthusiastic and flexible model suggests that those within a mentoring relationship need to be personally matched – individual tailoring to suit both parties. Whether those within the relationship should select each other or be chosen by a third party may also prove to be a contentious issue within clinical supervision. There could be a danger of collusion as well as the potential for reciprocity, and the advantages and pitfalls of choice in clinical supervision will be developed in Chapter 8.

Mentorship schemes have demonstrated a range of comparative problems; their degree of effectiveness has depended upon individual motivation, sufficient resources, selection and training, to name but a few. Burnard (1988) has highlighted the matching repertoire of skills required by a mentor to fulfil their remit, emphasising particularly the important attributes of a supporter: skills of active listening and empathy. Although the aim is to foster the mentoree's ability to discover and use their own talents, Burnard (1988) has also highlighted the role modelling function implicit in the role and the assimilation by the mentoree of elements of good practice.

New practitioners from pre- or post-registration courses need specific guidance and support in their transition, additional practical help with adjustments to practice as well as broader educational additions to their developing knowledge and skills in this new arena. Some will require more authoritative monitoring and assessment to ensure that standards are met. This is the main difference from clinical supervision, which needs a more delicate balance between the authoritative and facilitative approaches.

Clinical supervision refers more to an exchange between practising professionals, in which there is far less of a power divide between clinical supervisor and supervisee than, say, between student and mentor, although there may be some recognition of seniority and experience. We prefer to see preceptorship, mentoring and clinical supervision more as a continuum (this has recently been endorsed by the UKCC 1996) rather than acting as appendages or substitutes for each other. They all need to provide a range of opportunities for guidance, learning and support which should reflect the different degree and complexity of the needs of practitioners at different stages in their career and development. Many of the issues covered in this book, especially the skills development section, are equally relevant to those engaged in preceptorship and mentorship as they centre on the skills and pitfalls of purposeful interaction common to all. There are some core similarities, such as the need for a nurturing and supportive relationship. The differences are more ones of emphasis in the educative and authoritative functions of respective roles.

Comparisons with peer support

Illustrations of good practice in peer support undoubtedly exist (Holland 1987); many more have been highlighted in the initiatives of the National Association for Staff Support. However, problems with peer support have been endemic within the NHS (Booth and Faulkner 1986). Despite clear guidelines existing (Bond 1991), many have petered out through lack of structure, ideas, facilitation, group skills, leadership or just motivation. Blame has been fairly evenly directed at management or peers. Clinical supervision offers the potential for more structure, clarity and boundaries than many of the more unstructured support mechanisms that have limped on ineffectively or have petered out. It also serves to endorse the principle of support within the fabric of the organisation rather than leaving it open to the enthusiasm and energy of a few. However, as Swain (1995) reminds us, the support provided by clinical supervision is different from that which can be experienced within effective staff support groups, counselling and therapy services, and should never replace these services. They are needed now more than ever and should sit side-by-side with clinical supervision networks.

It is now important to explore some of the overt and covert driving forces towards the development of clinical supervision in nursing to understand why it may be interpreted so diversely. Many different viewpoints and motives propel its implementation. We need to look at some of these key influences, both those from other professional groups outside nursing and earlier attempts to implement a form of clinical supervision within nursing; we will then seek to identify further influential driving forces from within nursing.

External influences: what we can learn from other professions about clinical supervision

Many clinical supervision models being developed in nursing draw on the theory, development and experience of supervision in other disciplines. Many nurses themselves have had experience within these other professional groups, leading to them being strong advocates for clinical supervision within nursing. This impetus has been vital, but nursing needs to be wary of accommodating models in their entirety as they are built out of different professional philosophies and cultures. We need to select or adapt some of their component parts to fit our own professional orientation and organisational culture. (See Table 1.2.)

Table 1.2   What we can learn from clinical supervision in other professions

	Psychotherapy and counselling	Social work
Features	Built into professional culture and structure: compulsory for students, expected for newly qualified psychotherapists and counsellors, compulsory for all practising BAC-registered counsellors, most experienced psychotherapists continue throughout career	Built into professional culture and structure
		Useful buffer between field staff and management
		Immediate intensive backup in acute situations, without stigma
	Considerable emphasis on surfacing and learning about the unconscious processes which help and hinder the work with the client, including those of the therapist/counsellor	Widespread dissatisfaction may stem from lack of skills training and the power differential: supervisor is usually the supervisee's line manager
	Emphasis on building the 'internal supervisor' skills of the counsellor/therapist (i.e. in-depth self-monitoring and self-appraisal)	
Learning points	Aim to build into structure and culture, possibly making clinical supervision compulsory	Allow flexibility so that a supervisee can receive more clinical supervision sessions in acute situations, without stigma
	Develop the self-awareness element of clinical supervision by using structures and methods, not just vague rhetoric	Ensure supervisor is not supervisee's line manager
		Ensure adequate skills training for supervisees and supervisors

Psychotherapy and counselling

The term clinical supervision originally stems from the training and practice of psychotherapy (including psychoanalysis) and counselling. Trainees in these professions are expected to have weekly supervision for their work with clients, and some may be required to have two clinical supervisors during the training period. After qualification and registration, many continue with at least one clinical supervisor on a weekly basis and even the most experienced of practitioners would be expected to seek supervision for specific cases or emergent difficult clinical issues. The British Association for Counselling code of ethics (BAC 1993) insists on weekly supervision for all practising counsellors registered with them. Clinical supervision is built into the counselling and therapy culture; it is a prerequisite not a choice.

Supervision in this context is as much about the therapist/counsellor as the client. It not only focuses on the 'inner' and 'outer' world of the client and on clinical techniques within the therapeutic relationship, but also on the conscious and unconscious processes of the practitioner, their prejudices, blind spots and inner difficulties. The alliance between clinical supervisor and supervisee is analogous to that in the so-called 'therapeutic alliance' between therapist/counsellor and client as many of the dynamics being tussled with clinically in practice may resurface in supervision. This allows for some of the more hidden dynamics in the practice-based relationship to be focused on in the present and so enable a clearer understanding of what is really going on. The clinical supervisor may support the therapist/counsellor just as they try in turn to provide what is often referred to as a 'holding' environment, for the client to explore emotional difficulties and blocks to understanding and feeling. Supervisory support is also needed to help therapists/counsellors to 'work with the unknown' or to stay with the state of 'not knowing' (Casement 1985); this may also have important lessons for many nurses, who may have become too controlling or directive in their role. Casement's (1985: 19) influential work on the 'internal supervisor' – building the therapist's skills in self-monitoring and appraisal – may also resonate for those keen to see clinical supervision promote professional development and accountability in individual practitioners in nursing.

Many of the functions of clinical supervision in therapy/counselling have parallels in nursing. Nursing is essentially about relationships, with both clients and colleagues, and there are similar needs for practitioners to develop self-awareness and interpersonal and emotional skills to cope with the often stressful nature of their work. Swain (1995) suggests that clinical supervision in nursing could provide a similarly containing and holding environment – what Winnicott (1991) called the 'facilitating environment' – and so contribute to the lessening of professional anxiety and defensiveness. As Faugier (1992) warns, however, this approach in unskilled hands or, rather, unskilled mouths could so easily become intrusive or exploitative and lead to relationship 'traps'. She also suggests that this might lead to a confusion between 'therapy' and 'clinical supervision'. It would indeed be inappropriate if this were to happen in nursing, yet there tends not to be a confusion between these two distinct yet related areas in psychotherapy and counselling. Nevertheless, what is required in nursing is at a very different depth and intensity, especially regarding the highly complex world of unconscious motives. But to deny and devalue their application to clinical supervision in nursing is perhaps more dangerous than trying to adapt and use some of these 'relationship dynamics' from supervision in therapy and counselling. Nursing literature includes many references to the need to develop more self-awareness – easy to write and rather more difficult to do – in order to help practitioners delineate clearer boundaries between themselves and others, to see the difference between their own needs, motivations and wants and those of others. The human capacity to distort where oneself ends and another begins is notorious – almost as notorious as the human's capacity to deny that this happens. Hopefully clinical supervision in nursing can help provide this relatively 'safe space' to nurture practitioners' capacity to disentangle the complexity of their interpersonal relationships, whilst not losing sight of their wider professional principles and clinical aims.

Social work

Clinical supervision has a long history in social work, although it has often been supervision based on casework rather than a process which embraces some of the broader principles outlined earlier. Although some supervision focuses on the best allocation of resources for client groups, Hill (1989) suggests that it is more to do with providing the 'cornerstone' of professional practice and emphasises its role in improving the therapeutic proficiency of social workers. She also makes the point that supervisors act as a 'buffer' between social workers on the ground and those in management, which Butterworth (1992) suggests might also be a useful function within nursing.

Although Woodhouse and Pengelly (1991: 236) acknowledge that social services have a tradition of regular supervision, certainly when compared to health care, they suggest that 'it is commonplace to find that this has either lapsed altogether or become an arena for anxious case management rather than for reflective understanding'. Brown and Bourne (1996) write about the 'wholly inadequate preparation for this skilled task of supervisor' (in social work) which their book is designed to redress and refer to a range of research studies which highlight widespread dissatisfaction with supervision. They are quick to point out that excellence does exist and that the task is to encourage others to emulate those examples that work well. However, they also add a note of caution:

> Some of the dissatisfaction with supervision is structural and inevitable, stemming from the dynamics of a relationship in which power is not distributed equally and which also provides a focus for the wider frustrations and anxieties that arise in the daily, often stressful and demanding work of practitioners in social work and community care services.
>
> (Brown and Bourne 1996: 6)

Practitioners from nursing who have worked closely with social workers in families where there has been abuse, or where social needs are many and complex, have envied their social work colleagues' access to supervision whether ideal or not. As we implement our own models of clinical supervision, we can learn from these social workers who have had such a head start in the implementation of supervision systems. We should heed these messages about felt and actual power in supervisory relationships, and acknowledge that extensive good practice in supervision is dependent upon the coordination of effective training.

Given the type of culture we have in nursing we could look for further learning points from the established systems of clinical supervision within our own field.

Influences within nursing, midwifery and health visiting

Clinical supervision has been in existence in midwifery, mental health nursing and branches of the profession dealing with child protection (mostly health visiting and paediatric nursing). There are lessons to be learned from these early developments, and we need to take into account the culture of these contexts, in comparison to the culture of psychotherapy, counselling and social work. (See Table 1.3.)

Midwifery

Supervision has been an integral part of midwifery practice since 1936 when the role of inspector of midwives was changed to that of supervisor. The supervisor of midwives is designated by a local supervising authority and Bent (1992: 7) suggests that she is a key worker in the implementation of a principle which is at 'the very heart of supervision – the safety of mother and baby'. The route to this safety appears to embrace a specific model of supervision which links it firmly to managerial supervision and emphasises standards, accountability, professional misconduct and the legislative framework, all of which are clearly very important. Supervision in midwifery is often felt to be more of a management tool for staff appraisal and disciplinary procedure. This very singular version of supervision has been challenged both inside and outside midwifery, and the UKCC's guidelines (1996) implicitly deter others in the broader sphere of nursing from following this approach.

Others have been more explicit in their criticism:

The role [supervisor in midwifery] however has not developed into one of empowerment or professional development; rather one of guidance and direction to ensure practice is correct. It is also used to discipline when practice goes wrong. One would not wish to see clinical supervision within nursing and health visiting developing in this way.

(Briefing document on clinical supervision: HVA 1994: 4)

Midwives, like those within other specialities within health care, may feel themselves to be incompatibly different from colleagues in nursing and thereby indifferent to such criticism. Indeed the history of their own legislative framework has fuelled that difference. Yet concerns over the way clinical supervision has been translated exist within midwifery itself. The tension between those who wished to promote more of a growth and support model and those who insisted on maintaining the managerial directive approach was witnessed during the development of the controversial 'professional development' module, in material aimed at the preparation of supervisors (ENB 1992, module 4). The organisational emphasis is clear:

As we have seen whilst the supervisor is specifically concerned with safe practice and clinical competence, the manager is concerned with broader organisational goals such as the overall quality of services and the effective use of resources . . . The manager's interest in professional development is . . . a means of improving current performance at work and of making the most effective use of immediate human resources.

(ENB 1992: 16)

It goes on to suggest that Individual Performance Review is a tool which can help identify these staff development needs. This may not necessarily augur well for the principles of creativity, growth and support suggested earlier in this chapter.

Table 1.3　What we can learn from early developments in clinical supervision in nursing

	Midwifery	*Child protection*	*Mental health nursing*
Features	Long-established as management supervision, to ensure safety of clients by guiding and directing to ensure practice is correct Linked to disciplinary procedures Early recommendations that supervisor is 'counsellor and friend rather than relentless critic' have not been enshrined in the structure and practice of supervision and therefore lost	Policies require Trusts to have in place management monitoring of child protection procedures to ensure safety of children by guiding and directing to ensure practice is correct When managers are the child protection advisors, they tend to take over child protection work and become overloaded Child protection advisors who do not have a line manager role seen as being more effective	More contact with psychotherapy/counselling models of clinical supervision Long accepted as a concept, not widely established in practice Often with some inappropriate confidence that clinical supervision is 'old hat' Active use of structured reflection skills in supervisees often under-developed Support and catalytic skills often not well developed in clinical supervisors
Learning points	Hopeful statements about the growth and support element of clinical supervision are not enough: they need to be backed up with structures to ensure they are incorporated Other branches of nursing have similar cultures to midwifery and are therefore also likely to lose the growth and support element of clinical supervision if it is linked to disciplinary procedures Need for separate management monitoring and clinical supervision	Need to separate management monitoring of child protection procedures and clinical supervision	Need for re-evaluation of clinical supervision in areas where it has been established Not to assume that clinical supervision is happening effectively in areas where the concept is well accepted Be alert for any tendency to inappropriate psychotherapeutic interventions Ensure adequate skills training, even for those apparently experienced

Other branches of nursing have similar cultures to midwifery and are therefore also likely to lose the growth and support element of clinical supervision if it is linked to management monitoring and disciplinary procedures.

It is, however, interesting to note that in the preface to this material in Module 1, Bent (1992: 7) reminded us that a Departmental Committee in 1929 had recommended that: 'an inspector of midwives should be regarded as the counsellor and friend of the midwives rather than a relentless critic ... and make them feel that there is always someone to whom they can look for sympathetic understanding'. However, these sentiments seem to have been mislaid during the intervening years.

The current predominant language of service requirements and 'resource commodities' overshadows the human needs suggested in this early document in midwifery, and since then endorsed by the UKCC as being essential for the implementation of clinical supervision in the rest of nursing and health visiting. We can learn from this that hopeful statements about the growth and support element of clinical supervision are not enough: they need to be backed up with structures to ensure they are incorporated as central to the process of clinical supervision.

We hope that those supervisors of midwives who would like to balance their supervisory contact by developing more of a professional and support component to their role will find the rest of this book useful, and that it could bolster rather than dilute the unique statutory and professional aspects of midwifery practice.

Child protection

The uneasy alliance of clinical supervision and management supervision is not unique to midwifery but has existed in a more limited way in specific areas of practice such as child protection work. For many community practitioners, clinical supervision is totally associated with managerial supervision for child protection but this is only a part of the role, for many an extremely small part, albeit a stressful and anxious one. In areas where child protection numbers are higher, some have already questioned the logistics of this system as well as the narrowness of its focus and approach. The reviews of key child abuse cases (Department of Health 1991a) and the document related to the Children Act (Department of Health 1991b) have led to policies requiring managers to ensure regular review and monitoring of all aspects of work in this context. Parkinson's (1992) study of her own local policy in the London borough of Tower Hamlets led her to challenge its effectiveness:

> The impossibility of carrying out this policy without excessive management workload ... precipitated a management crisis ... The policy document also seemed to be one step further towards restricting and controlling community nurses, rather than enabling, empowering and supporting them to take professional responsibility for their own work.
>
> (Parkinson 1992: 41)

She also challenges the Department of Health's guidance to senior nurses on supervision in child protection work. She raises important points about whether line managers can meet the full supervision needs of community staff who are working with abusive families and whether a line manager can provide a safe environment in which to discuss feelings about child abuse.

This experimental study, which compared earlier manager-led supervision with the extended supervisory function of new child protection advisors who had no managerial responsibility, found the personal and professional benefits of the latter to be enormous. She also suggests that it was felt to enhance the individual's own responsibility and accountability: 'Some staff explicitly contrasted this with the situation before the project, commenting that they felt managers took on, or took over, responsibility for child protection work once they had been brought into contact with it ... One manager also thought that a large number of staff felt "safer" in their work' (Parkinson 1992: 49).

This example again supports the premise, endorsed by the UKCC, that the line manager should not undertake the role of clinical supervisor for those staff for whom she holds management or disciplinary responsibilities. As Swain (1995: 40) states passionately: 'Any moves to establish links between clinical supervision and formal disciplinary process should be challenged. This is not to say the two should never touch. Clinical supervision is integral to good management which in turn is integral to an effective, healthy organisation'. Both the need for clarity of separation of management–supervisor roles, and the need to communicate with and integrate into managerial systems, will be addressed in Part III.

Mental health nursing

Presumably due to greater links with the worlds of therapy/counselling, the concept of clinical supervision has been part of mental health nursing for some time. White (1990) and Ferguson (1992) suggest that clinical supervision is more developed among nurses working in psychiatry, particularly in community settings, and yet as Thomas (1995: 27) has candidly admitted, 'it is indeed a very mixed bag' and it may be happening to some extent in some areas but certainly not in others. This is also emphasised by Carson *et al.* (1995: 54): 'Although the concept of clinical supervision is well accepted in mental health nursing, it is a less well established reality for most practitioners. It is clear that clinical supervision is certainly not yet the norm for the majority'.

Our experience in workshops has tended to support this view, where there is a tendency for some mental health practitioners to show a rather bored 'been there, done that' attitude. Yet it is clear within the skills component of the courses that many aspects of clinical supervision have often been poorly thought through and practised (with some outstanding exceptions). The tendency to over-'therapise', pathologise and use non-responsive listening or interpretations by way of support is also more apparent in this group than in others. As a result, many supervisees we have observed have been (understandably) defended against the self-disclosure required for in-depth reflection on practice. Faugier's (1992) warnings of inappropriate therapeutic interventions may need to be heeded. Our observations indicate that skills assessment and training are necessary for many experienced supervisees and clinical supervisors. The experience of clinical supervision for mental health nurses highlights the need for re-evaluation of clinical supervision and the need not to assume that clinical supervision is happening effectively in areas where the concept is well established.

The explicitly espoused aims of established clinical supervision systems could be viewed from the perspective of the professional cultures in which they are situated. Psychotherapy has explicit emphasis on valuing the 'therapeutic use of self', along with in-depth reflection on oneself and the part one's own personal qualities, abilities and feelings play in the professional care of the client. There is little or no managerial monitoring of psychotherapy practice

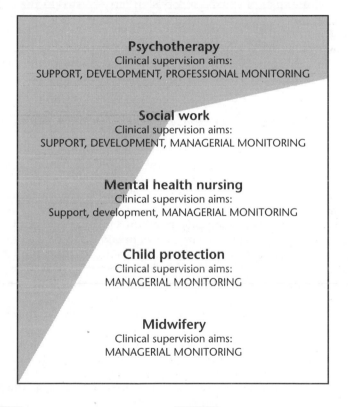

 Explicitly valuing therapeutic use of self as part of the professional culture

Explicitly valuing management monitoring as part of the professional culture

Figure 1.2 Main aims of clinical supervision related to various professional cultures

since most of it is done outside institutions and it is impossible for managers to observe practitioners at work. Social work also has a degree of explicit valuing of 'therapeutic use of self', but within a definite (and necessary) managerial structure for monitoring practitioners, which tends to increase standards of procedural safety but inhibits the development of 'therapeutic use of self'. Mental health nursing has some degree of explicit valuing of 'therapeutic use of self', within a management monitoring system. Child protection in nursing has less explicit valuing of 'therapeutic use of self' and even greater explicit managerial monitoring, while midwifery has very little explicit valuing of 'therapeutic use of self' enshrined within the culture, with considerable emphasis on managerial monitoring. Notable exceptions do exist in these nursing examples whereby explicit valuing of 'therapeutic use of self' coexists alongside rigorous managerial monitoring. However, we are taking a broad general view here. Figure 1.2 highlights these comparisons.

So, specific examples of clinical supervision have existed in the profession for some time but all of them either offer a limited vision of its potential or have been inconsistently implemented. More recent developments have made it imperative for all practitioners and their managers to adopt more extensive and better thought-through systems of clinical supervision within their organisations. The last part of this chapter will briefly describe this.

The impetus for clinical supervision from within nursing

Recent developments have provided the impetus for clinical supervision to become an urgent agenda item in any discussions and projects aiming to sustain and develop nursing practice. These developments include: broad organisational changes; policy directives; concerns about accountability; quality initiatives for improving standards of care; concepts of empowerment and partnership becoming integrated into nursing philosophy; educational drives towards reflective practice; concern about practitioner health and preventing burn-out; and increased value placed on therapeutic interventions and concomitant requirements for self-awareness. We wish to celebrate and emphasise these positive factors which are pushing the nursing profession towards developing clinical supervision. However, in this section we also point to some of the ambivalence which can block this development and upon which we expand in the next chapter.

Some of the principles pushing factors for clinical supervision are outlined in Figure 1.3, forming the first part of a force field analysis diagram. We will complete this force field analysis in Chapter 2 by examining the blocking factors which have so far impeded and may continue to impede the effective development of clinical supervision in nursing.

Broad organisational changes

Health care is becoming increasingly complex and more demanding of everyone. Technological change is only one part of this. Much of it is due to extensive change within the organisational structure of the NHS and in the

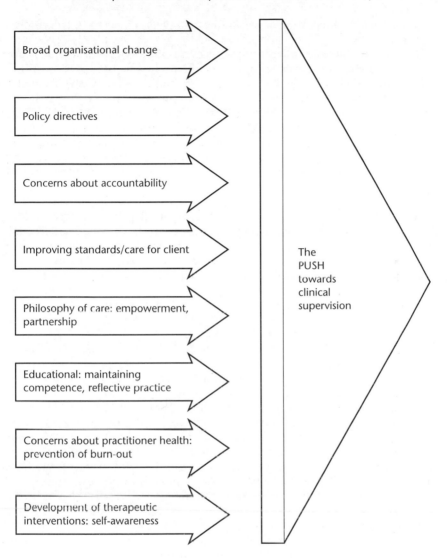

Figure 1.3 Factors which have contributed to the present impetus towards developing clinical supervision in nursing

philosophy of health care provision, with the impact falling heavily on clinical nursing staff. As Swain (1995: 14) puts it: 'Repeated organisational changes tax even the most flexible of practitioners. Continuing clinical work while at the same time practising creatively through the development of imaginative ideas for future practice requires professional stability, boundaries and containment.' There is increasing recognition that clinical supervision can be a system for providing this stability, boundaries and containment to enable practitioners to cope with and positively adjust to organisational changes.

Although at the time of writing the election of a new government means that some of the issues covered here may themselves be the focus of further change, the previous Tory NHS reforms have had an all-pervasive influence on prevailing NHS culture. The NHS and Community Care Act 1990 radically altered the entire structure for organising and financing care in both the acute and community services. Unlike previous reorganisations, which had little direct impact on everyday care and treatment, these changes have had unprecedented influence on how all practitioners deliver care to patients and clients, and how they themselves are managed. The demands of the internal market and the relocation of power and management in the National Health Service has put pressure on every single practitioner to rethink how they perform their work, and how they must skew or adapt their priorities. Purchasing contracts with commissioning authorities have to be adhered to. Future contracts depend on it. And yet practitioners who are closer to client groups have often had little say in the early negotiation of contracts and have seen the quality of their health care interventions sacrificed for quantity. Many initiatives exist to encourage practitioners to develop the necessary skills of marketing, skill mix and campaigning to influence purchasing decisions (HVA 1994; Department of Health 1994), but the 'marketing' language and skills are alien and alienating for many.

The internal market has become even more complex in the community with the controversial 'wild card' role of GP fundholders. Norman (1993) suggests that because they have the ability to buy cheaper community services from elsewhere (some have bought from geographically distant Trusts), this both destabilises local Trusts as well as disrupts and fragments established working relationships. It is also very confusing for clients. She does, however, clearly refer to the advantages of fundholding too, which she suggests relate to the potential for more integrated team work and more speedy access to health care for their own practices. However, if some have preferential access, others will be having to make way for this access, and one of the biggest criticisms of fundholding is its capacity to produce a two tier system of primary care and so heighten the notorious growing divide in health inequalities. The Community Care part of the Act has also been subject to extensive criticisms in all client groups. Its honourable rhetoric about caring for people in their own homes has not been matched by the resources to do so (King's Fund 1997), leaving community practitioners at the very sharp end of care. Greater numbers are being discharged earlier so one set of colleagues meeting targets puts increasing pressure on others.

As Watkins (1993: 436) has said, 'Community care should be a philosophy not a place'. Sadly it is often viewed more simplistically and pragmatically as a place – a cheaper place. The main carers here of course are not even community practitioners, but those who have always provided the bulk of care in the community – families and carers, and usually women. Wynne (1994) and others have recorded how community care policies have placed an additional burden on women carers. As the majority of our nursing work-force are women this may place a dual burden, professional and personal, on them too.

The Patient's Charter (Department of Health 1991c, 1993c) has made more promises than the resources given to match them. Although most practitioners would heartily agree with the new complaints procedures introduced to challenge shortfalls in service provision, many do feel that they have been left to face understandably angry and upset clients with both hands tied behind their back, unable to offer the services that grand mission statements have promised to provide.

Inequalities in health care continue to exist and their nature is changing, with greater awareness in the nursing profession about their impact. Although the Tory government (1979–97) vociferously denied the mounting inequalities in health care, both national and local reports have highlighted these increasing inequalities based on poverty indicators: Townsend and Davidson (1982), Whitehead (1987), Jacobsen *et al.* (1991) and Blackburn (1991, 1992) focus on class; the reports of Chevannes (1991) and Ahmad (1992) highlighting race. Some of these inequalities affect not just client groups 'out there' but many practitioners in nursing who in turn may become recipients of health care; we are all potential clients.

Racial and sexual inequalities are mirrored particularly well within the layers of the employment hierarchy, despite attempts to address equal opportunities in the workplace. Such attempts include a *Programme for Action* (Department of Health 1993b) to increase numbers of ethnic minority staff and *Opportunity 2000* (Department of Health 1991d) to increase very low numbers of women in leadership positions (Rafferty 1993). Many believe there to be a mismatch between rhetoric and reality in the development of equal opportunities. Robinson (1992) argues that some developments in nursing, notably in primary nursing, actually serve to reinforce sexual and racial divisions. The new Labour government has now made a commitment to address inequalities in both access to, and delivery of, health care.

The restructuring of management has led to the virtual obliteration of nurses within Trusts and there are very few in purchasing positions. This has led many nurses to feel under-represented and marginalised in negotiating crucial decisions for service provision. The flattened management structure in nursing has put pressure on the role of team leaders to provide this leadership and to implement the changes, whilst still fulfilling their clinical responsibilities without additional resources.

Skill mix, where it has been done with full involvement and negotiation of staff, has resulted in a better utilisation of appropriate skills all round. But it has often been implemented solely with cost cutting in mind, more 'what grades do we choose to afford?' rather than 'what skills do we need to meet the health needs in our speciality?' Lightfoot *et al.* (1992) and Cowley (1993) have challenged the financial as well as the clinical effectiveness of some of these poorly thought-through and cynical 'value for money' exercises. Ironically, although buffeted by all these organisational changes which increasingly affect the way practitioners think, make decisions and prioritise their work, many say that direct contact remains the same, insomuch as people are still scared and vulnerable when ill, carers still want the best they can get for loved ones, babies still assert their right to be born and cared for. This makes for growing tensions between the demands of the client and the sometimes conflicting demands of employers. Clinical supervision is needed not only to help practitioners cope with the pressures of all these many changes, but also to enable them to face the ethically demanding nature of some of these tensions and the ensuing dilemmas. The clinical supervisor may herself feel that she is in the centre of a triangle of often competing demands – those of the practitioner, the organisation and the client. She needs to have the skills and resilience to work with the clinical dilemmas that emerge. In today's National Health Service the clinical supervisor is required to have an understanding of the needs of both the provider and the purchaser and of nurse and client.

Clinical supervision is not only essential for the individual during this pace of change, but it is vital for the organisation too. Johnson (1995: 23) states that:

> the consequences of poor or absent supervision for the organisations can be serious. These include decreased accountability, poor or restricted performance, a high incidence of staff turnover and sickness, staff burn-out and resistance to change. Supervision gives real clarity without which collaboration cannot function effectively.

She goes on to cite some particularly dire consequences of poor collaboration in the community in child abuse case reviews (Department of Health 1991a).

Policy directives

Although there has been a growing professional impetus towards clinical supervision, it required political endorsement to give it additional potency and weight. Policy directives ensure that clinical supervision will become a national concern rather than left to areas of good practice. Although in the short term this may mean that the implementation of clinical supervision in some areas is based on compliance rather than commitment, and may be interpreted and introduced in a minimalist way, the directives nevertheless provide an essential long-term lever to improve clinical supervision systems.

A Vision for the Future (Department of Health 1993d) was the first document officially to recommend that the concept of supervision should be explored and developed: so that it is integral through the lifetime of practice, thus enabling practitioners to accept personal responsibility for, and be accountable for, care, and to keep that care under constant review. It mirrored the UKCC's emphasis on the parameters of safe practice and the educational requirements for greater professional autonomy and accountability within the Scope of Practice (UKCC 1992b) and the potential extension of this practice, when it announced that it 'is central to the process of learning and to the expansion of the scope of practice' (Department of Health 1993d: 15).

In its much-anticipated position statement on clinical supervision for nursing and health visiting, the UKCC (1996) suggests that clinical supervision should assist all practitioners to develop a deeper understanding of

Table 1.4 UKCC's (1996) key statements about clinical supervision

1 Clinical supervision supports practice and aims to maintain and promote standards of care
2 Is a practice-focused professional relationship to assist guided reflection
3 The process of clinical supervision should be developed by practitioners and managers according to local circumstances. Groundrules should be agreed so that practitioners and supervisors approach clinical supervision openly, confidently and are aware of what is involved
4 Every practitioner should have access to clinical supervision. Each clinical supervisor should supervise a realistic number of supervisees
5 Preparation for supervisors can be effected using 'in-house' or external education programmes. The principle and relevance of clinical supervision should be included in pre- and post-registration education programmes
6 Evaluation of clinical supervision is needed to assess how it influences care, practice standards and the service. Evaluation systems should be determined locally

what it is to be an accountable practitioner in the context of the realities of clinical risk management. They emphasise the potential organisational benefits to be accrued from this, linking to the NHS Executive six medium-term priorities for 1996–7: 'to develop NHS organisation as good employers with particular reference to workforce planning, education and training, employment policy and practice, the development of teamwork, reward systems, staff utilisation and staff welfare' (UKCC 1996: 3).

The UKCC places clinical supervision firmly in the context of the profession's need to develop lifelong learners and makes an important assertion (UKCC 1996: 3) that 'Clinical supervision is not a managerial control system' and thereby should not be hierarchical in nature. The UKCC's Position Statement includes six key statements which can be found in summary form in Table 1.4.

Concern to improve standards of care for clients

Although many initiatives in nursing have been motivated by a desire to improve client care and service delivery, it is also sadly true that clients may become lost behind grand professional posturing and a plethora of theories and concepts. We would do well to be reminded that: 'The first principle of clinical supervision must be that clients should benefit, individually and corporately, directly and indirectly' (Swain 1995: 22). Standards of care need to be at the root of clinical supervision. It is about what we do for our clients, how we listen to, talk to and relate to clients, what the outcomes of our contact with them are and what the overall clinical effectiveness is. It is about efficient and effective use of our time. Maintaining and enhancing standards needs to be placed and viewed in its political and social educational context, and the centrality of client care in the organisational and educational context has been at the heart of all continuing education initiatives (UKCC 1993).

Changing philosophies of care: health, partnership, empowerment

The last 20 years have witnessed a gradual demedicalisation of nursing and a slow maturing of nursing as a profession moving away from a training and practice based on the biological/medico-sciences towards ideas from sociology, psychology and educational theory. The growth of notions of nursing independence, epitomised by process-based nursing, has resulted in related emphasis on individual autonomy and accountability which, some suggest, have left many practitioners adrift between theory and the shifting sands of clinical practice, without some of their defensive mechanisms of the past. Butterworth (1992: 5) suggests that models of clinical supervision can be developed which will offer some protection 'giving nursing the necessary support it needs to mature into greater independence'.

Movement towards a more person-centred approach has led to demands for patient advocacy rather than direct intervention and for working with clients in partnership, aiming to empower rather than 'do to or for' or 'talk at or about'. The move towards health promotion and prevention even in the acute branches of nursing, albeit slow and incomplete, (*Making It Happen*, Department of Health 1995) has challenged us to retreat from crisis ad hoc responses and reflect on the possible range of long-term choices, encouraging the essential involvement and participation of clients en route. For Faugier (1995) clinical supervision and patient empowerment are very closely linked. Yet despite the numerous advantages of working to involve and empower rather than control, outlined by many commentators and practitioners such as Pearson (1988) and Chavasse (1992), this shift in approach presents a threat and a challenge to the practitioners who are reluctant to let go of time-honoured ways of relating professionally (Bond and Holland 1992). Kendall (1991) is one of many researchers who have found that working collaboratively with clients is more of a myth than a reality even when practitioners earnestly believe that this is what they are doing. There is a need to disentangle the realities of working in partnership from the more superficial rhetoric associated with the term; its true implications for both client and practitioner could be teased out within clinical supervision. There is increasing recognition that the true development of partnership and empowerment requires the kind of backup support and challenge provided in the clinical supervision relationship.

Concerns about accountability

The UKCC's Code of Practice, and related guidance on the concept and practice of accountability from the initial *Exercising Accountability* (UKCC 1989) to the current *Scope of Professional Practice* (UKCC 1992b), have all challenged practitioners to focus on maintaining clinical standards and to link this with the growth and development of their own competence and educational progress (UKCC 1993). Professional accountability is, however, only one aspect of legal accountability. Dimond (1990) highlights the different types of accountability when she compares and contrasts it with accountability to the client, to society as a whole, and to the employer.

Although to maintain accountability in one arena may automatically ensure accountability in another (for instance, accountability to clients based on confidentiality is part and parcel of our professional accountability outlined by the UKCC in the *Code of Professional Conduct* (UKCC 1992a)), many dilemmas in practice can result from a clash between professional account-ability and accountability towards an employer (Holland 1991). Pressures on Trusts to curtail and limit resources can have both a direct and an indirect impact on the ability of individual practitioners to maintain even their current scope of practice. Practitioners need help and support to clarify the implica-tions of the many-faceted nature of accountability in everyday practice and there is increasing recognition that clinical supervision can provide a forum for this.

In an increasingly complex organisational picture of different multi-disciplinary settings, there is also a related growing need for clarity about roles and the boundaries between individual practitioners, especially when philosophies and approaches to client care, needs assessment and service delivery may clash. Shifts in power in some employment partnerships in the community, such as those suggested in *Primary Care: The Future* (Department of Health 1996b) as well as the controversial shifts heralded by the extended role of the nurse and skill mix, all demand a shrewd grasp of accountability principles in practice. As Johnson (1995) has suggested, clinical supervision can allow for the development of role clarity without which teams cannot collaborate effectively.

The actual process of clinical supervision may on occasion also provide a challenge to the clinical supervisor's practice of accountability. We have endorsed a non-managerial approach to supervision, but there is much con-cern about what happens when it is clear to the clinical supervisor that the supervisee's practice is not 'good enough' and may even be unsafe. (This is looked at in the section on clinical supervision contracts in Chapter 3.)

Developments in education

There have been both direct and more subtle changes in educational philo-sophy and approach in nursing, shifting away from control of the content of clinical material to encouraging ownership by learners of their own educa-tional process. The emphasis is more on *how* people learn, on encouraging a diversity of learning styles and needs, and on achieving a better educa-tional balance between authoritative and facilitative teaching styles. It has been important to encourage safe, experiential learning (Kolb and Fry 1975) to allow for an emotional and personal engagement with the theory. This approach to adult education is more likely to encourage practitioners to take responsibility for their own 'lifelong learning' and to use clinical supervision as part of this. The UKCC's (1993) requirements for education standards reflect the commitment of nursing, midwifery and health visiting to this idea. However, for many teachers and learners, these have been painful shifts. Once again there is a reluctance to let go of much safer scripts, to focus on regurgitating the 'what' rather than asking why, and to be more directed and directing than enabling in its broadest sense.

Reflection has become one of the key 'buzz words' of educational theory and practice since Schön's influential work in the 1980s (1983, 1987) and it is intended as a tool to attempt to bridge the divide between theory and practice. Many different models have been devised and some are selected and adapted in Chapter 3 as frameworks to guide and supplement reflective thinking. However, there is a growing awareness that value placed on it in the nursing literature is not always mirrored in practice. Swain (1995: 9) suggests that: 'We speak and write of reflective practice, yet experience out in the field suggests a very different reality. Time for reflection is in fact a very rare commodity indeed.'

Increasingly, the profession is seeing that clinical supervision may offer just such a forum for space and reflection. This 'reflective space' could also help practitioners to integrate theory to practice, increase awareness of research findings and help develop practitioner curiosity and confidence.

Evidence of the importance of paying attention to practitioner health

Evidence of the advantages of promoting supportive cultures in the workplace abound. Cooper's (1981) and Hingley *et al.*'s (1986) work refers to the economic and efficiency benefits to the organisation in the form of reduction in sick leave and reductions in the mobility and attrition of the workforce. Butterworth *et al.* (1997) suggested that nurses were experiencing a time of increasing stress levels in the 1990s, as compared to other projects carried out in the 1980s using the same measure, the Nurse Stress Index. They also found from using standardised instruments that clinical supervision could stabilise and in some cases reduce these measurable stress levels. In their work on preceptorship (but equally relevant when applied to clinical supervision) Morton-Cooper and Palmer (1993: 31) suggest that: 'if we can become more understanding and supportive of our colleagues, then similar values could be carried in our day to day work and help us to communicate more fully (and perhaps more honestly) with those people who place such faith and trust in us at times of crisis and transition in their lives'.

Swain (1995: 29), humane as ever, reminds us that practitioners need help for themselves first and foremost, before they can be of help to others: 'We need to take our own grief and stress somewhere, express it and deal with it'. Johnson (1995: 22) also refers to the managerial and organisational benefits of clinical supervision; she states that it could help practitioners develop 'their emotional responsiveness so that they don't become burnt out and so that they remain able to offer a high quality service in a climate of rapid change'.

Swain (1995) suggests that some of the low priority given to strategies that might aid emotional support or give time to reflect is due to the realities of a very pressured external world which results in practitioners marginalising their own physical and emotional health. She and many others suggest that the impact of the tremendous organisational changes brought in by the 1990 NHS reforms (especially the commercial ethos of the internal market, and what many experience as an anti-clinician climate) adds to this stress, and carries with it a devaluing both of the clinician and the clinical work. In the early 1990s there were many draconian statements alluding to the percent-age of sickness rates in nursing, offering harsh remedies to rectify them, all rather Dickensian in tone. This non-compassionate culture is not unique to nursing. There has been a vibrant anti-professional political culture in the 1980s and 1990s in many diverse service professions such as education, social work, probation, police and prison services, and many have shared similar feelings of resentment and loss, resulting in low morale and attrition of the workforce. The nursing literature is full of references to 'support' and the need for nurses to develop more emotional skills, yet self-care has not in general featured highly in the nursing agenda, nor is it truly just a product of more recent political change, although this has undoubtedly exacerbated it. Lip service is frequently paid to the need to support each other but the lack of extensive support networks indicates the poverty of both organisa-tional and individual commitment to them.

Increasing value placed on self-awareness as a therapeutic skill

When the work itself is intrinsically highly charged and makes emotional demands, and when this is added to by the pressures of rapidly changing organisational demands and limited resources, there is a need not only to offer more extensive structures for support but also to encourage individuals to build their own skills in survival and growth. The current push towards helping nurses increase their self-awareness is essential if nurses are to look after themselves more and contribute to a healthier, more caring workforce culture. Self-awareness will also allow for more sensitive and effective inter-ventions in their work with clients and improve clinical standards and care. It will improve our capacity to help ourselves and others.

Yet Guggenbuhl Craig (1971) reminds us that our unconscious drive towards helping others can in itself lead to unhelpful ways of being and relating. Heron (1990) refers to these as degenerative interventions and you will be exploring many of these pitfalls throughout the skills chapters of the book. Much of Hawkins and Shohet's (1989) work on supervision focuses on the concept of the 'wounded helper', which we shall explore in the next chapter, and although they rightly suggest that our 'wounds' or vulnerability can be a strong asset if recognised and supported, they can also lead to uncon-scious interventions that are not helpful to others or ourselves. Therefore our capacity to understand, respond effectively and to help is more likely to be genuine, appropriate and centred in the client if tempered by understanding of ourselves and our motivations.

As Hawkins and Shohet (1989: 5) state: 'our experience is that supervision can be an important part of taking care of oneself, staying open to new learning, and an indispensable part of the helpers on-going self develop-ment, self awareness and commitment to learning'. This links to the need to build your own 'internal supervisor' (Casement 1985) which can be used in reflective learning in practice and brought back to your actual clinical super-vision session for further honing, clarification and help. In this way we can learn to watch, listen to and understand ourselves as well as our clients and so 'stand back' from the relationship to assess and monitor it as well as take part in it. This is not the same as being emotionally distant or aloof from another or from ourselves, but it is a way of building inner resources and awareness to improve and develop our work.

Well thought-through and resourced systems of clinical supervision could indeed help meet many of our own unmet professional needs, which are both a part of these forces pushing for change as well as a by-product of some of the more positive forces. All practitioners need an uncontaminated, supported and supportive space to share, reflect and analyse what they do and how they feel. This will provide a focus for developing skills for effective practice, so contributing to improvements in practice. However there is also a great danger in viewing clinical supervision as a universal panacea for existing shortfalls or ills. It will be as effective as the commitment, training and resources allocated to it, and to the skills and compassion practised in the clinical supervision relationship. Chapter 2 presents the other side of the coin already identified within the ambivalence of some of the 'push' factors in this section. It explores some of the more resistant elements to this change and focuses on the vital emotional underpinning of clinical supervision.

2

The hidden picture: resistance to clinical supervision and implications for the clinical supervision relationship

Although the momentum towards implementing clinical supervision has been growing in recent years there is also concern about why it has taken so long to become accepted in nursing and how it can really take root and grow in a culture that can be so resistant to major change, particularly change which is dependent upon encouraging closer professional relationships. Undoubtedly there is sufficient political will to support it in principle but it remains to be seen how extensively and effectively it will become an organic part of nursing life and be truly instrumental in helping support and develop clinical practice.

Maybe during your reading of the first chapter you also felt your cynicism rising as the old mantras reappeared. Don't we know enough already, you might think, about the need for accountability, for working in partnership, for improving standards of care? We are all trying to survive great organisational change and have been for some time. Prevention of burn-out through developing self-awareness has been acknowledged for more than 20 years so why are we still going on about it? The repeat button seems to be stuck. And yet we are all destined to keep on repeating ourselves, both individually and collectively as a profession, until what is being aimed for is felt to be understood, accessible and attainable.

This cannot happen until the powerful processes which inhibit us from understanding and reaching our perceived wants and goals are also acknowledged, accepted and understood. In so doing we can divest them of their power to sabotage the process and identify more realistic ways of being effective. We have to bring the unacknowledged and therefore unknown unconscious processes between ourselves and others, be they clients or other colleagues, into our awareness; we need to bring them to the surface where they can be seen and coped with more easily. Similarly we have to understand that within the organisational culture we may also be affected by the unconscious processes belonging to the organisation as a whole, which although are not directly part of us, can still impinge on our capacity to work in the way we would like to, and can confuse and distort how we ourselves act and think.

All of this is part of the crucial emotional underpinning of clinical supervision and indeed all human relationships. But this is particularly important in a professional supervisory relationship which espouses the principles of growth and support and centres on reflective practice as a way of improving the care of ourselves as well as of our clients. Towards the end of the last chapter you explored the factors influential in 'pushing' towards clinical supervision. As a means of counterbalancing this we will start with an overview of the forces within ourselves and the organisations in which we work which will unconsciously try and resist this major force for progress and change. We will then link this more directly to the implications for the clinical supervision relationship and types of unconscious communication that can take place within it. From this we will distil some of the practical implications for developing clinical supervision to allow for its valuable potential to mature rather than wither.

Resistances to clinical supervision

Although the potential value of clinical supervision is extolled, the literature is also full of anxiety and misunderstandings about it. Some of these anxieties have real components to them; pressure on time, staffing levels and resources are factors of life in the NHS and will have an impact on the frequency of, and commitment to, clinical supervision. And yet many nurses have always used these factors defensively to avoid thinking about and applying aspects of professional change. Given the history of defensiveness in nursing, it is not surprising that clinical supervision may be viewed with suspicion.

Clulow (1994) refers to the ambivalence generated by the term and the fear of either being overly controlled or nannied – 'We were struck by the negativity about supervision' (1994: 181), resulting in lip service being paid to the need for it, without any real conviction or active commitment to it. Platt-Koch (1986: 7) has said: 'confusion about and resistance to clinical supervision could be depriving nurses of one of the most valuable tools in existence for learning and refining skills of assessment and treatment of patients'. Hill (1989) suggests that practitioners tend to think of their supervisors as authoritarian and that the whole concept of clinical supervision is linked conceptually to an authoritarian figure. Hill goes on to decry this 'because clinical supervision is much wider and generous in its intention' (1989: 9). Fear of being disempowered in the clinical supervision process led community nurses from one neighbourhood nursing team, in Kohner's (1994) overview of clinical supervision in practice for the King's Fund, to reject the concept. They preferred to describe what they received as advice, support and

professional guidance rather than clinical supervision. Although their reluctance to embrace the term may be understandable, their reason for doing so
is more worrying. They seemed to want to protect their own autonomy and
control over particular areas of practice and expertise: 'it feels uncomfortable
and threatening to have someone supervise you. Most community nurses
have picked this sphere of nursing to get away from control and lack of
autonomy over their own practice' (Kohner 1994: 31). Clinical supervision
is clearly seen here as a critical intrusion rather than a positive relationship.

Both individual and organisational defences may serve to block the establishment of clinical supervision and/or be destructive to its effectiveness
once established. These resistances, rather like many of the push factors in
Chapter 1, interlink with each other and it is difficult to see where one
begins and another ends. They impact on and leak into each other, and yet
each has distinctive characteristics and roles to play. We need to ask what
they are protecting us from and why?

The simple question to ask to start with is why do we need to defend
against clinical supervision? We develop defences as protective devices to prevent us from feeling anxious but this anxiety tends to mask other deeper feelings. They serve to protect us in particularly difficult situations when we feel
we have to be seen to cope. Yet both these individual and collective defence
strategies in nursing have also led to ways of working and relating that are
counter-productive to effective practice and personal emotional survival. The
protection they give is flawed and may actually cause a range of other problems. Coping defensively (and often ineffectually) is very different from
developing and using skills to manage and contain our anxiety when we
both need and choose to. Then we are more in control within the situation,
rather than unconscious defence mechanisms being in control of us.

In clinical supervision this continuum of resistance, moving from deeply
defended to accepting, is shown in Table 2.1. The more hidden underlying
feelings that the defences are trying to protect from are also outlined. We
need to explore these components in more depth.

First, we will enlarge on the types of defences in nursing, and relate some
of these more specifically to clinical supervision and then we need to identify the main anxieties they are protecting us from, which, for simplicity, we
will take from Figure 2.1 (see p. 49) and divide into:

- fear of personal and professional power, of inequalities in power, and the
  impact of this on our own skills and autonomy
- fear of developing more secure, supportive working relationships and professional attachments
- the fear of emotions and expressing feeling – leading to a pervasive anti-
  emotional climate.

If you were to place them opposite the push factors in Chapter 1 you might
be forgiven for thinking that in logical and practical terms the push factors
would have a 'walk-over'. However, Lewin (1972), in his model of force field
analysis which seeks to compare the comparative influence of factors affecting change, warned against such an assumption. He suggests that the resistant factors which spring from our feelings, even though we may be unaware

Table 2.1   Levels of resistance to developing clinical supervision

Individual nurse

1 Rejection – 'get enough criticism and interference from management as it is'	2 Irrelevant to me – 'good idea but too busy'	3 Resignation – going through the motions	4 Give it a try – tentative testing the water	5 Commitment

Organisation

1 Rejection of the real principles – just rename IPR or management by objectives as 'clinical supervision'	2 Irrelevant to us – 'too costly'	3 Resignation – paying lip service	4 Pilot projects	5 Commitment

Hidden issues

1 Struggle for power, control, autonomy	2 Fear of relationship	3 Fear of emotional floodgates opening	4 Interest, relief	5 Valuing, seeing effect on practice

of them, can undermine a greater number of factors which stem from apparent common sense and rationale. The factors which allegedly make 'no sense' can be much more powerful than ones which do. How do we make sense of these hidden forces?

Anxiety and defences

Individual and collective anxiety

Anxiety is part of the human condition. How individuals respond to anxiety is at the root of much relational research. It is central to managing internal and external conflict. It determines the way we feel about ourselves and how we interpret our experiences. It provides an important alarm system to alert us to situations that we will find stressful. Appropriate and realistic anxiety can be a spur to creativity and growth. However if, in our early histories, anxiety is not contained by another (as it is in good enough mothering), or we are not helped to contain it at other times throughout life, and if we in turn do not learn to use it as a resource, then the internal conflict it produces becomes unmanageable and it works against us. We are then compelled to bury or block it, but still acts as an 'undercover agent' to distort our perceptions and actions, leading to inappropriate or limited responses. The role of anxiety in organisations and the social defences that arise from it has long been acknowledged to have a major impact on behaviour and attitudes in the workplace. Anxiety increases when the level of risk is perceived to be high, and sturdy social defences may grow to protect or anaesthetise us from these risks. The factors that determine how you identify sources of risk, and assess the degree of this risk will vary. They may evolve from your own history of handling anxiety, the role and degree of responsibility, authority and power you may feel you have in your professional life, and both the overt and covert strategies that are employed in the organisation to include or exclude, control or motivate others. There is an interplay between organisational and individual anxiety and defences: 'we see organisations as key sites where early anxieties are replayed; and we see the very structures of the organisations as reflections of the apprehensions and frustrations of their members. Organisations are emotional arenas' (Fineman 1993a: 30–1).

The health care organisation is a particularly emotional arena where Menzies (1959), in her influential work on social defence mechanisms in nursing, spelled out some of the strategies through which this interplay was enacted. For Menzies these defences develop over time as the result of collusive interaction and agreement, often unconscious, between members of the organisation as to what form they shall take. The socially constructed defence mechanisms then tend to become an aspect of external reality to which old and new members have to adapt. For instance many enthusiastic students or returners to practice, with their imaginations fired by the potential of nursing practice, often have to face the reality shock (Kramer 1974) of colleagues who have defended themselves by becoming cynical and disinterested. How they too may subsequently inherit the habitual ways of reacting and defending is well expressed by Obholzer and Roberts (1994: 9) 'Newcomers may be able to see more clearly but feel that they have no licence to comment. By the time they do, they have either forgotten how to see, or have learned not to. They too require defending against their anxieties, not the least the anxiety of upsetting their colleagues'. Although Menzies' (1959) original study is now fairly old and only focuses on hospital nursing, much of it is as depressingly relevant today as it was then, and her more recent work alludes to this (Menzies Lyth 1988). Some of the specific examples within the defences have changed but others have replaced them. We need to acknowledge that many specialities in nursing have worked hard in both their education and practice to shift some of the more task-oriented, ritualistic, and emotionally distant behaviour and explore the value of engaging more openly and directly with the raw emotions implicit in their contact with clients. The most obvious examples for this are within the hospice movement and in work with people with HIV and AIDS.

Social defences

Menzies referred to the following defence mechanisms, which determined the culture and shape of the organisation of nursing work, and protected the nurses from the anxieties that threatened to overwhelm them. We have enlarged and added to some of them. See how relevant you think that they are to you in your area of practice. You may have to make a distinction between the current jargon of intended practice versus the reality of practice:

- keep the nurse and patient apart as far as possible as it is the closeness of the relationship which increases anxiety. She cited task orientation, rotas and compulsive paperwork as methods for achieving this
- depersonalisation – patients are labelled, and categorised, often linked to an illness or problem. The contribution of emotional life, family context and social environment is ignored
- the rhetoric of coping and detachment – a defensive 'don't care' attitude, 'a good nurse must not get too involved', 'nurses should always cope'. Menzies emphasised how attachment needs are minimised not only between nurse and patient but between nurse and nurse, referring to the lack of stable, consistent working placement and the practice of moving nurses around wards to fill in gaps
- checks and counterchecks to reduce the weight of responsibility about ultimate decision making about a patient
- rituals – repeated tasks, lists, non-individualised questions and procedures
- repression, discipline and reprimand – a whole chorus of critical feedback responses which result in a reluctance to seek feedback. This links to a fear of making mistakes, leading to an emphasis on 'playing safe' rather than using initiative
- collusive social redistribution of responsibility, leading to projections of blame and irresponsibility onto others
- responsibility and accountability avoided and pushed upwards to avoid fear of retribution. This minimises the exercise of discretion
- avoidance of change
- obsession with tasks, making it difficult to prioritise; difficulty letting go of time-honoured approaches in order to try something new
- the ultimate detachment of leaving the service: 'it is the tragedy of the system that its inadequacies drive away the very people who might remedy them'.

(Menzies Lyth 1988: 79)

We would like to enlarge briefly on how some of these defences may be replayed in our current climate and mention others which we have witnessed frequently within accounts about anxieties about clinical supervision (see Figure 2.1). They may refer both to direct client care and to work with other colleagues (the potential content of clinical supervision sessions) as well as to the nature of the clinical supervision relationship itself and include the following.

- Being immobilised and stuck, blocking all suggestions for moving on. There is a strong resistance to problem solving or even to thinking. We may block and parry all suggestions – with 'we've done that, it doesn't work'. We may emphasise how awful it all is and repeat it endlessly. Many of our actual complaints may be more than justified but we then defend ourselves from the hurt and the loss of feeling unsupported, misunderstood and generally unacknowledged by others and then feel disempowered to do anything about it.
- Avoiding the inevitable discomfort of learning about new things which may include recognising our current limitations in some areas. Anxiety

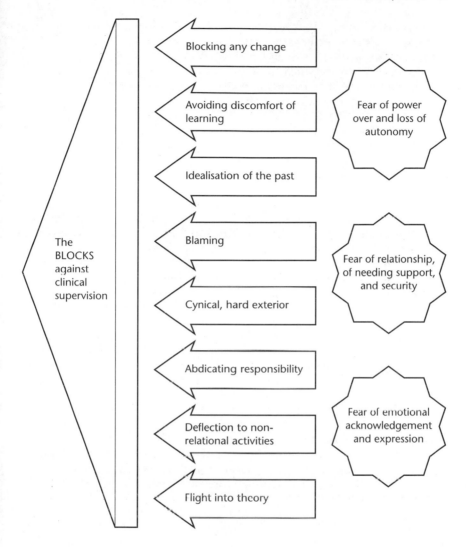

Figure 2.1 Defences which block the effectiveness of clinical supervision and the unacknowledged fears behind them

may often be a block to learning, and part of the task in clinical supervision is to enable those involved to test their perceptions in the light of new possibilities. For example, a senior ward manager may be asked to develop some new skills so that she can supervise others. She may feel defensive at first, but given the opportunity to express and discuss her fears, may begin to value the opportunities for new learning that preparing for role change provides. Others may defensively cling to their years in practice as proof of their experience and the non-necessity of doing additional training. We forget that unless we learn from experience, mere length of time in practice may be meaningless.

- Idealisation of the past or different ways of working: for instance, some older nurses may be stuck in the myth of the rosy idealisation of their own youth and of nursing-as-it-was, as a defence against the reality of adjusting to changes and perhaps against the sorrow of loss of their own youth. Woodhouse and Pengelly's (1991) study of anxiety within a group of health visitors referred to their idealisation of more 'expert' agencies in dealing with specific problems, and the corresponding diminution of their own sense of personal competence and authority.

- Projection of everything that is felt to be wrong onto something or some-one else. All the 'bad bits' of our working lives, and the conflict that they arouse, are the fault of someone else – management, other nurses, other multidisciplinary colleagues. To deny that these feelings of conflict reside within us, and to protect ourselves from all that is bad, we have to defend our own righteous position and ensure that the boundaries between 'us and them' are made more and more rigid and impermeable. Woodhouse and Pengelly's (1991) work, which explored the adverse effects of anxiety in working collaboratively in partnership between a range of agencies in the community, refers to the poor collaboration that results from such 'toxic conditions' and to the condemnation and intolerance that can accompany it. This can lead to feelings of being victimised – 'the world is against me' – and of being an innocent partner in the whole mess.

- Hiding feelings of loss, shame and guilt under a cynical and harsh exterior. This can lead to an apparent rejection of moral considerations, where another's feelings become irrelevant to personal or organisational survival. This again is visible in the 'dog eat dog world' of competition and marketplace survival.

- In order to defend against fear of getting it wrong, making mistakes and not knowing, some people may divest themselves of responsibility for both the process and outcome of their work, preferring to follow in the slipstream of another. A supervisee, for example, may expect their clinical supervisor to do all the work involved in setting agendas and later follow-through of action. It is easier for some to sink into apathy rather than run the risk of imagined failure or inadequacy.

- Deflection or displacement of attention onto a component of work which is less risky and which thereby allows us to distance ourselves from the real source of anxiety (often linked to attachment relationships). The flight into paperwork and bureaucracy is an example of one such distraction technique. Some deflective strategies, whilst giving an impression of being very busy, actually result in sabotaging any real involvement with the main task or tasks.

- Flight into theory – to protect ourselves from engaging in real emotional understanding, in which we can tap into our own experience and empathy to appreciate what might be being experienced by someone else. It can feel comforting to focus on intellectual understanding. We were once asked to review a book on stress in nursing which managed to cover more than 200 pages without once mentioning how it feels to be anxious and stressed.

There can be a similar tendency for some practitioners to focus on endless models of clinical supervision to avoid thinking about how to implement supervision realistically. Casement (1985: 4) suggests that 'Theory also helps to moderate the helplessness of not knowing' and thereby is an attempt to reduce anxiety, but goes on to remind us that 'it remains important that this should be the servant to the work . . . and not its master . . . By listening too readily to accepted theories, and to what they lead the practitioner to expect, it is easy to become deaf to the unexpected'. This principle is echoed within an excellent guide on measurement and evaluation tools (Campbell *et al.* 1995) which challenges us to not devalue the totality of our work with clients by being restricted by the current climate's narrow demand for quantitative outcomes, but asserts instead the importance of being open and responsive to unintended contacts and outcomes in the evaluation of our work. They admittedly focus on work in the community where unintended outcomes are particularly relevant amidst the complexity of community contacts, and where initial object-ives have to be modified to meet more immediate and pressing health needs.

Many readers will either have direct experience of the social defences first described by Menzies or recognise that some elements of them still flourish today, but along with the intervening years has been a growth in those who have challenged and tried to rework some of this unwanted inheritance. Many practitioners in our workshops state that they feel devalued by the social system and deprived of personal satisfaction, and want to exercise their full range of skills with more creativity and responsibility. Many recog-nise that their capacity for care and concern, compassion and empathy, and for action based on these feelings, the fuel for their initial motivation to work in nursing, has been hampered by these defensive restraints and that the protection they offer is often neutralised by the dissatisfaction and ero-sion of confidence that they bring. They also recognise that blaming the 'system' is one way of prolonging the feeling of helplessness and that col-laborative action to change some of the restrictive practices does work. Let us hope that clinical supervision can provide a forum for this.

Fears about power and autonomy

Initial fears about, and therefore resistance to, clinical supervision are often related to a sense of having to lose control over what you do, of feeling oppressed by having to fit clinical supervision into an already busy schedule, or worrying that, by its very nature, it will involve another person (the supervisor) invading your work. The clinical supervisor tends to be viewed as a figure of authority and often can be an authority figure in reality, if only by virtue of seniority rather than having a management role. We need to tease out both the real and imagined aspects of power issues in clinical supervision and how they manifest both interpersonally and within the structures of the organisation. Broader inequalities in the manifestations of power in society, in the form of gender, race and sexuality, may impact on both of these. It is interesting too that power is often viewed as 'bad' or abusive; there is little room for positive images of authority and influence implicit in having power in nursing, and we wonder how this affects a nurse's capacity to enable, encourage and empower.

Reality of power structures in clinical supervision

Undoubtedly not all the suspicious or protective feelings leading us to resist clinical supervision are solely to do with being defensive or being unable to focus on the positive attributes of clinical supervision. There can be very real, justifiable issues around the use of power in clinical supervision, related to how it is managed within the service or how it is conducted within the working alliance of clinical supervision. Brown and Bourne (1996: 32–3) suggest that

> It is this structural dimension of power that is frequently understated and underestimated in its impact on the clinical supervision relation-ship . . . These personally, culturally, structurally and institutionally based inequalities of power . . . will have an effect in addition to, and interlinked with the more obvious power issues associated with the relationship between a clinical supervisor and a supervisee.

Sources of individual power in clinical supervision

Having 'power over' rather than 'power to' within a professional relation-ship has a very different feel to it. Drawing on Kadushin's (1992) different components of power, let's see how it might relate to clinical supervision in nursing and identify when it might be deemed to be controlling rather than enabling (see Figure 2.2).

Designated authority

Agency – the power to influence

Access to learning resources

Personal attributes

Figure 2.2 Sources of the clinical supervisor's power – the emphasis
Source: Adapted from Kadushin.

Kadushin distinguishes between four main sources of power:

- *Designated authority* – implicit in the position/role of supervisor. As we are explicitly advocating that clinical supervisors are not also the supervisee's line managers this may help to reduce the confusion over status and authority that the merger of these dual roles can bring. Although for many this merger of roles might enhance and legitimate the supervisor's authority, it can also lead to some confusing messages about how the power of the clinical supervisor may be used. It could easily emphasise the normative aspects of the role and allow for a rapid shift into areas of coercion and retribution, and possible disciplinary procedure should certain organisational criteria not be met. The midwifery supervisor has a clearly legitimated normative function within her role. This makes the 'power over' function much clearer and many other Trusts and Units would like to see this principle established in other areas of nursing practice. Some supervisors, of course, who do not have legitimated permission to pursue this aspect of the role will delight in a more controlling and authoritarian stance even when this approach is not intended in the Trust. In contrast to this, the UKCC (1996) has essentially supported the more formative and restorative functions, preferring to emphasise the need to develop the 'power to' be more effective and accountable, rather than 'power over' to ensure this. The clinical supervisor can still have 'designated authority' but this is reflected more in respect for her seniority, experience and skills. Even though the clinical supervisor may try and promote the latter enabling and collaborative image, some supervisees may not be able to get past their stereotype of the more authoritarian and controlling image of the term 'supervisor'. Whatever power stance is adopted there needs to be clarity about what is to be done if clinical standards are not being met (see Chapter 3).

- *Agency* – the clinical supervisor has the power to influence a supervisee to do something or behave in a certain way. This may involve a more controlling approach involving coercion or the offer or withholding of rewards. A clinical supervisor choosing a more encouraging and self-directed approach may suggest or make recommendations for further training or a move to another post. Each approach may also include the covert 'reward' of negative or positive feedback respectively, thereby seeking to restrict or motivate supervisees.

- *Resources power* – Handy (1990), writing about managers within organisations, regards this as the most important and potentially influential source of power at one's disposal, in order that change can really be effected. It is more difficult to see the sorts of resources that supervisors have the authority to use, which is perhaps the main disadvantage of divorcing it from the management role. Sometimes 'power over' resources can be very enabling! However resources do not necessarily have to be economic resources, but may also relate to sources of knowledge and ideas which can be encouraged and shared.

- *Personal attributes* – this may include the force of personality, energy and enthusiasm of the supervisor, and the skills and experience they tap into in their role as supervisor. This may include some aspects of modelling which may be positive or not. For instance, a charismatic and dazzling personal style can unfortunately lead to disempowering the supervisee. These personal sources of power also belong to the supervisee, of course, and the sharing of aspects of experience, skills and personal attributes can lead to mutual exchange and respect for what each has to offer. In Kadushin's (1992) study in the USA, focusing on perceptions of power in the clinical supervision relationship, both supervisors and supervisees found that positional and personal power were the most relevant. Perhaps you might like to reflect which components best sum up your feelings about where power, in its broadest sense, may lie within your own clinical supervision relationship, and whether its use enhances or depletes your own professional abilities.

Structural power

Attributes of individual influence and power need to be placed in a cultural and organisational context to appreciate additional layers of covert power implicit in the relationship. For instance how might gender difference affect the relationship; how might it feel to have a clinical supervisor who is white in a practice workforce that is predominantly black? A thorough overview of the complex and important issues related to discrimination/anti-discriminatory practice and oppression and anti-oppressive practice is covered by Brown and Bourne (1996). Although their work refers to social work practice, which has a longer history of training and action in inequality issues, it is just as relevant to health care, perhaps even more so as there is a dearth of anti-discriminatory training throughout the layers of the service. The Department of Health's (1991d) response to the Opportunity 2000 initiative attempted to address the lack of women in senior positions at all levels of the National Health Service first highlighted by Salvage (1985) in the 1980s, although the NHS organisational reforms appear to have increased rather than tackled the problem of gender disparity in positions of influence and power. As Davies (1995) reminds us, it is the masculinisation of the whole culture that is even more relevant than statistics related to gender/professional status, in the inequality debate (more of this later in the chapter).

Ahmad's (1992) work on the politics of race and health highlights the social and health status inequalities in the delivery of health care in this country, and the ethnocentric bias and discrimination in mental health are well addressed by Fernando and colleagues (Fernando 1995). These inequalities are mirrored in the workforce profiles in health care and in the comparative paucity of black and ethnic minority staff at senior levels. Increased emphasis on the need for anti-discriminatory practice for both client groups and colleagues has increased over recent years (Department of Health 1993b) but there is still a marked lack of training for anti-oppression/discrimination for practitioners.

During recent years, the Royal College of Nursing has supported an increased awareness of inequality factors affecting gay and lesbian staff: concerning visibility, openness, acceptance and trust, the comparative need for a reduction in prejudicial, homophobic responses to lesbian and gay clients and their partners. These deficits and inequalities must be tackled structurally by employers, translating anti-discrimination laws into more proactive commitment to action.

How might these wide and complex structural dimensions of unequal power relationships impact on clinical supervision? The clinical supervisor needs to be aware of their own prejudices and assumptions which might distort the time and attention given to the supervisee, and the way the organisational structure may contribute to disparity. They may need to acknowledge the realities of difference, but seek to ensure that the person is treated equally and fairly (avoiding collusion in an attempt to over-compensate) whilst at the same time recognise some of the additional blocks and hurdles they may have to overcome to be accepted and effective in their role. The supervisee may in turn be adversely affected by racist, sexist or homophobic reactions from clients and need support in dealing with this. The supervisee, of course, may harbour discriminatory thoughts and attitudes about the clinical supervisor, which may also affect their commitment to the process. But we have focused more on the potential effects on the supervisee, as the clinical supervisor may be perceived to be, or is in, the more authoritative position, and this may enhance felt difference.

Interpersonal aspects of power

Our personal feelings about and behaviour towards people in positions of perceived power often stem from our own childhood experiences, however far away and distant and faded they may seem. Throughout childhood, adult carers exercise enormous power over children and the types of attachments engendered can create lifetime patterns for the way the future adult will relate to others in an authority role. These patterns of course are not immutable; they can change through experiencing and internalising different ways of relating and so shift our perceptions of how we are 'allowed' to be with another 'parental' figure. But some patterns can be enduring, especially at times of stress (see attachment patterns later in this chapter for a fuller account of this) and this can lead to transferring our images from the past onto an authority figure in the present.

If the clinical supervisor represents authority in some way for you – and this will be compounded if there is a managerial component to this role and if your experience of authority figures from the past was that they would try and undermine or even demolish you – then you might only focus on certain comments or feedback which seem to you to be critical, dismissive and authoritarian. The term supervision, as Clulow (1994) has suggested, may itself be instantly translated by some into an image of an authoritarian relationship even before the real people in the relationship actually meet each other. Assumptions may be formed and critical projections directed towards the other. These critical projections may take many forms. The other person may be seen in a variety of negative forms – as useless, unhelpful, not trustworthy; they may arouse envy or competition. They may be seen as too 'mumsy', stifling and suffocating, encouraging you to withdraw in order to find your own independence. Conversely if there is a pattern of idealising authority in the past, then they may be imbued with equally inappropriate ultra-positive projections – they may assume an all-knowing guru status, always knowledgeable, always right, which leaves the supervisee always infantilised, always looking up to the supervisor. Whether feelings about the authority figure are negative or positive the result is similar – the supervisee can be stripped of their own authority and confidence.

Reality of personal power in role of supervisor

Brown and Bourne (1996) suggest that supervisors in social work are not comfortable with their authority and power and seek to side-step it. We would endorse that this is very much reflected in nursing in a great many aspects of the role. Nurses often deny the authoritative dimension of their work and role and are over-diffident when faced with the professional authority of another. There often appears to be a deep confusion between being authoritative and authoritarian. Heron (1990) makes a strong distinction between these two different concepts, which may have the same root but differ substantially in how they might be received and accepted in the long term.

- *Authoritative*: refers to the authority you have by virtue of the experience, knowledge and skills acquired in your role and in your development. You may assert this 'authority' when you feel it is appropriate to do so with varying degrees of emphasis depending on the wants or needs of the recipient. You still respect the other person, encourage collaboration, include their views and perceptions and support their right to make up their own mind and not agree with you. You can admit when you do not know and that some things are not 'knowable'.
- *Authoritarian*: means that you are absolutely sure that what you say is right, based on an expert-knows-best approach. You do not acknowledge the right of the other person to make up their own mind or allow for disagreement. You are really seeking compliance. Sometimes an authoritarian approach may be packaged in the guise of the former but the evidence of the need for control and compliance and the lack of collaboration seeps through.

The authoritative approach tries to encourage a more collaborative, symmetrical relationship based on encouraging 'power to' rather than 'power over'. If the clinical supervisor believes in the support and growth model of clinical supervision rather than just endorses organisational norms, then the clinical supervision process has to be interactive rather than one-way and should be compatible with the principle of empowerment – can in fact put the 'power' back into empowerment and so endorse and encourage the confidence and autonomy of the supervisee.

The over-use of this term has been critiqued by Salvage (1992), who suggests that the move towards professionalisation and creating nursing experts may just replicate the older power relationships that doctors had with their patients, this time nurses assuming the mantle and the emotional distance that goes with it; that they need instead to let down their restrictive all-knowing barriers and work more collaboratively with clients. Skelton (1994: 417) adds a touch of cynicism about the misuse of 'empowerment' – 'it is essentially about getting you to come round to a way of behaving that I the expert knew in advance was good for you, whilst encouraging you to think that changing your behaviour was your idea in the first place'. This is a salutary reminder for the clinical supervisor with her supervisees and for the practitioner with her clients. Salvage (1992) goes on to remind us that if we are to empower clients then we do need to empower nurses but not to give them power to use over clients. The clinical supervision relationship could help model this difference.

Power, autonomy and the supervisee

If the clinical supervisor is more comfortable with establishing an interactive, collaborative relationship without the abuse of power, then the supervisee's own professional confidence and accountability can develop. Again this is more easy to imagine happening within a clinical supervision relationship which does not have a managerial component.

As Brown and Bourne (1996: 34) remind us, a symmetrical rather than asymmetrical power relationship in clinical supervision can enable:

- recognition of the clearly defined limits of the legitimate power of the clinical supervisor
- understanding that this power is to be exercised constructively in a two-way relationship between people of equal status and worth as human beings
- recognition of just how much the supervisee has to contribute to the working alliance in clinical supervision.

We would add

- the importance of both clinical supervisor and supervisee identifying their rights and responsibilities within the relationship and engaging in two-way feedback as a way of monitoring the process of clinical supervision (see Chapter 3).

It is sad that there is so much misunderstanding of this potential, so much resistance to it, and ways of relating that lead to the abuse of power rather than its constructive use.

The fear of developing professional relationships

Try as we may, it is difficult and, we would suggest, undesirable to divorce our 'external' professional self from the personal 'internal' sense of who we are and how we feel. Our early life experiences are a key to understanding the emotional resources that we have at our disposal in current working relationships. They can provide clues for some of the difficulties we experience in our contact with both clients and colleagues. Attachment theory, when applied to both individual development and the organisations in which we work, can offer a framework for understanding many of the insecurities that occur in working relationships.

In the last 30 years there have been two major developments in nursing practice which have been concerned with allowing closer human relationships to be part of the care of patients: open visiting on children's wards and the individualised patient care/primary nursing/named nurse approach for patients of all ages. In both cases, there was massive resistance in the profession against the introduction of these developments. Being more emotionally involved with patients would get in the way of all the essential tasks that had to be done. Yet now we would be shocked to find a paediatric ward with restricted visiting and which did not address the emotional, attachment and play needs of children; or an adult ward run on a task allocation system: we would consider these approaches as inhumane and detrimental to recovery. The development of attachment theory had a direct influence on changing attitudes and practice in paediatric nursing and, we believe, an indirect influence on increasing the relational component of the organisation of adult patient care. There is more acceptance that, whatever age they are, human beings need consistency and reliability in relating to other people and that this need is even greater when experiencing the trauma of ill-health when they are separated from those to whom they are attached. Therefore it might be fruitful to borrow some of its concepts to construct a framework for understanding the needs and resistance of nurses as regards clinical supervision.

Early attachment theory

The 'founder' of attachment theory was John Bowlby who, in his famous trilogy on attachment (1971), separation (1973) and loss (1980), suggested that attachment to others was an intrinsic biological human need, which was clearly visible in infancy and childhood but was equally relevant throughout the life span. He emphasised the importance of the child's emotional as well as physical needs and the sort of emotional environment necessary for good enough emotional development. He stressed the need for security and consistency, the need for sensitivity and responsiveness from parents and carers, in order to develop secure attachments that could weather the conflicts and losses that are part of all relationships. His early work outlined the problems that could occur for both individuals and for society at large if these basic human needs were not met and when the lack of a sense of a 'secure base' could result in a poor sense of self; more insecure, conflictual relationships with others; and potentially wider social problems of fragmentation, alienation and anti-social behaviour.

Bowlby's work contributed to James and Joyce Robertson's moving films about children in hospital and residential care in the 1950s, 1960s and 1970s and the long-term traumatic effects of poorly managed separation especially when combined with lack of consistency from alternative carers (Robertson and Robertson 1989). Although vociferously attacked by many doctors and nurses at the time, their work later led to important shifts in social and hospital policy. Perhaps it now seems so obvious to focus on the emotional needs of sick children and to ensure that parents can accompany them in their care that it is easy to forget how recently these changes occurred, and how strong the professional resistance to them was. Many still have problems in translating some of these principles to the needs of adults at times of illness and stress. The professional resistance to providing regular, consistent support for nurses through clinical supervision is an example of this. The potential impact of current attachment research on social institutions and social policy (Kraemer and Roberts 1996) is as relevant today as it was in the 1960s and certainly very relevant for life in large organisations.

Secure and insecure attachment

Attachment theory outlines the conditions in which the learning of social and emotional skills can most effectively take place. It is essentially based on the simple premise that those who are treated respectfully are more likely to be respectful to others, and that those who are cared for without being robbed of the sense of who they are can develop and grow and provide, in turn, non-intrusive, sensitive and appropriate care for others. Attachment theory can perhaps most clearly be seen in the early development of attachments between parents and children, and in the ensuing behaviour of children related to their internal sense of self. Under 'good enough' conditions the quality of these relationships becomes internalised (Bowlby's term for this was 'internal working model') and so coalesces into a coherent personality – someone who feels realistically good and confident about themselves.

Mary Ainsworth's pioneering work with families in the home and, later, in controlled research studies (Ainsworth *et al.* 1978) fleshed out Bowlby's work in early development and provided an important initial framework for highlighting the differences between secure and insecure attachments and types of insecure attachment. This early work has been extensively replicated in numerous samples, many testing its applicability to different cultures (Grossman *et al.* 1985; Miyake *et al.* 1985; Sagi *et al.* 1985). More recent in-depth studies involving intensive observation of infants with parents (Stern 1985, 1995) support much of the early attachment research and add to our understanding of how the development of that baby's internal sense of self is so sensitive to vicissitudes in the relationship with the main carer. Attachment research has also been widened and extended to include many longitudinal studies of children at different ages, and these have highlighted the long-term impact of early attachments on later relationships in childhood and on the child's skills in emotional expression and ability to get on with others. (See the Minnesota Studies from the 1970s to 1990s; Sroufe *et al.* 1990.)

Adult Attachment

Numerous extensive research studies on attachment in adults relate to the durability of many early attachment patterns, and their replication in adult relationships, both within patterns in their relationships with others and in communication with others. Mary Main's work in particular, in the Adult Attachment Interview (Main and Goldwyn 1985; Main 1994), provides clues for assessing the quality of adults' relational attachments. She focuses on how comfortable they are talking about adverse experiences, the inner conflict that can arise, and their emotional responses. One of the important outcomes of this work is that it demonstrates that those who develop some awareness and understanding about adverse experiences, those who can 'name them' and talk about them rather than block them off or become engulfed and enmeshed by them, can learn to deal with the conflictual feelings they produce. Attachment patterns are durable, but not rigid templates that are totally resistant to change. They can shift through developing more secure relationships with others.

In nursing, the bereavement studies of Parkes and others (Parkes *et al.* 1991) have been the most influential extension of attachment research in adults, adding to our understanding of separation and loss; but studies into more everyday expressions of adult attachment needs and loss are being developed all the time (Bartholomew and Perlman 1994; Sperling and Berman 1994). Attachment research has become a huge growth area and much of it is relevant to our work in health care and in understanding our own responses, as it spans the 'external' world of what is observable and 'said', and the internal world of major emotions and how we are really coping.

Attachment relationships and clinical supervision

It is important to remember that attachment research is not about categorising or labelling people, but that it provides a framework for understanding the effects of key relationships in a person's past and present. Attachment patterns can only be seen in the context of relating with others. Although durable, particularly at times of stress and anxiety, especially when linked to the fear of separation and loss, they are open to change. New ways of relating can be learned.

As clinical supervision is essentially about a relationship between two people, many of our own past ways of relating may be retriggered within it either through reactions of the supervisee's relationships with clients or within the dynamic of their own working alliance. It will impinge on all the feelings and reactions to power and authority explored earlier in this chapter. Those with more personal experience of insecure attachments may find establishing closer working relationships more difficult. Those with a history of predominantly insecure avoidant attachment may avoid close contact with others and even choose a speciality which allows for maximum independence. Others (those with insecure ambivalent attachment histories) may become more enmeshed with their clients or with their clinical supervisor but also resentful of the feelings of dependency this may lead to. Both clinical supervisor and supervisee may find it helpful to acknowledge the part their own personal history of relationships may play within their professional relationships, particularly at times of stress. It is also important to remember that those of us with the most secure of histories can be knocked sideways at times of acute stress or trauma, even though our capacity for recovery may be greater. In group clinical supervision, of course, these attachment relationships will be even more layered and complex, rather like they are in families. It is ironic that peer group clinical supervision is perceived as the 'easier option' in this context. It is only the resourcing of it which may be simpler.

Attachment in organisations

In order to make sense of the influence of attachment histories, we have concentrated on personal attachment relationships between people, but the overall professional and organisational culture can also enable or diminish people's capacity to attach and relate to each other in a meaningful way. The question you might like to ask yourself is – how well does your organisation provide a secure base for you to practise in? The notion of a secure base, first coined by Ainsworth (Ainsworth *et al.* 1978) and then developed by Bowlby (1988), does not mean an ideal environment, but one which provides a 'good enough' supportive context for individuals to explore, try things out and develop their skills and confidence. It develops an independence of spirit rather than dependency, feared by so many.

- Are consistent working relationships encouraged or positively discouraged?
- is time invested in building team work or is your team a collection of disparate individuals who squabble and compete with each other most of the time?
- are you consulted over major change policies or are they imposed on you?
- is there a climate of trust or of suspicion?
- are the main policies which frame your work consistent with the philosophy of your role or are they restrictive to that role?
- is a major change followed by a period of reflective review and consolidation or are too many changes happening at once?
- is there regular planned protected time for reflection on your practice that you can rely on?

Many of the major organisational changes in the NHS over the period of the so-called reforms have tended to heighten insecurity. The marketplace culture is one based on competition rather than cooperation. Some aspects of competition may well be healthy but they can also serve to alienate groups and individuals from each other, and can lead to coercion and threats in order to achieve targets. Many workshop participants have alluded to what seems to them to be the 'divide and rule tactics' within their units, leading to the splitting up of good working relationships and a reduction in motivation. Where there is insecurity there can be incapacitating anxiety and the pace of change of recent years has certainly tended to heighten both.

Confusion and distrust are also enhanced when people are asked to work in a culture of mixed and conflicting messages. The emphasis on partnership is a good example. Glossy mission statements in many Trusts allude to the principles of working in partnership. Many practitioners do desire to work in this way with their clients, but they find that the way they are treated in turn is the reverse of this philosophy. They often feel infantilised and controlled, rather than empowered to empower. Many are left deeply cynical about 'soundbite' management and the falseness and lack of congruence between mission statements and reality. More recent work on the political and organisational aspects of attachment allude to some of these discrepancies: 'The markets depend upon non-market institutions, on trust, on relationships between people and within communities, on norms of good behaviour, on social capital. Destroy that and you not only damage efficiency, you also destroy the conditions for a good life' (Kraemer and Roberts 1996: 1); and: 'A culture with a relentlessly competitive ethos undermines trust and maximises insecurity and it is hard to believe that this can be healthy for society, even in its economic relationships, in the long run' (Marris 1996: 194). Ironically it is the fostering of secure attachments, rather than the current compulsive drive towards angst and chaos in the NHS, which will facilitate the creativity, motivation, autonomy, accountability, efficiency and effectiveness needed in the workplace.

The need for a secure base

To hope for a major organisational shift from insecurity to security would be idealistic indeed, in the current climate. But perhaps the main message that we wish to extract from this overview of attachment is that clinical supervision could eventually attempt to provide, even in the most fragmented working environment, a space for stability, consistency and responsiveness. A relationship built on trust and support could provide the 'secure base' so desperately needed by everyone – an oasis amid the emotional aridity that is so often a by-product of continual change and confusion.

Attachment theory and its application do not provide all the answers to the complexities of both personal and organisational development, but the ideas within them, bolstered and strengthened as they have been by extensive and varied empirical research, have much to inform us of the way we relate to each other. They also provide an understanding of how and why more defensive patterns may emerge in relationships and why the emotional contact needed for security and support is feared and neglected.

Anti-emotional climate in the nursing profession

Faugier (1995: 8), in selecting a 'growth and support' model of clinical supervision, seeks to counter the lack of emphasis on the emotional effects of nursing work: 'I worked on the wards as a student nurse in psychiatry where people committed suicide and nobody ever discussed it. Nobody ever talked about what had gone wrong, what we should have done, and what we should have all been thinking. I know that still goes on in some settings. That was wrong and it has to stop.'

Nurses from all specialities have had to learn to keep their emotions under wraps. We have a history of creating stiff upper lips. We had to learn consciously how to apply aseptic technique to physical wounds, and unconsciously had to learn how to develop a parallel emotional asepsis to protect our wounds of vulnerability. Messy and wayward feelings must be prevented from contaminating our work. This analogy of linking emotions to the dangers of infection control has been developed by Dartington (1994), who explored the impact of contradictory beliefs in nursing leading to despondency, passivity and an avoidance of emotional attachment to others:

If for a moment, we consider the institution as the patient, it is as if emotional dependency is experienced as the most contagious of diseases. Everyone is under suspicion as a potential carrier, and an epidemic of possibly fatal proportions is likely to break out at any moment. The only known method of prevention is stoicism, which is administered by example and washed down by false reassurance.

(Dartington 1994: 105)

Many of course do acknowledge ambivalent or difficult feelings, but tend to develop personal strategies to deal with the stress they cause. Within the organisation as a whole emotions tend to be marginalised; there is seldom time to deal with them in ways which might help. In the King's Fund's exploration of the need for clinical supervision, Kohner (1994: 5) found that nurses did not have mechanisms to talk about successes and positive feelings let alone the feelings of uncertainty, inadequacy and despair that were commonly expressed. As one of them said: 'In nursing we are not going to get away from the bad things in life . . . it's what it's all about, to make those bad things a little more bearable for the people involved'. This nurse was referring to her clients, but emotional stress needs to be made more bearable for nurses too. We need to identify how the organisational culture contributes to the denial of emotions.

Organisational suppression of emotions

A great deal of work that has been done on understanding how organisations are structured and how people within them behave has ignored their essential unique human ingredient – feelings. If feelings have been referred to it has tended to be in the context of 'attitudes about' work rather than understanding how the organisational culture itself allows or disallows certain types of emotional expression. It often takes the form of a censor and, by pathologising certain forms of emotions, seeks to stifle them. Hearn (1993) and Parkin (1993) link this to the fact that, in political terms, organisations are masculine arenas where emotions are seen as feminine, uncontrolled and irrelevant or even dangerous to achieving the main task. However, women, usually of lower organisational status, are often used to deliver 'bad news' and deal with the aftermath of negative emotions. Putnam and Mumby (1993) harness the concept of 'emotional labour' to suggest that our emotions in organisations have been controlled to a far greater extent than is normally recognised. They explore how some emotions may be selected for use and incorporated as commodities for instrumental ends. For instance, a climate which encouraged wariness and fear holds potential dissidents and challengers in check; professional accountability may encourage whistle blowing to reveal poor standards but employees are often silenced and disempowered for fear of losing their jobs. They suggest that this is not only pernicious for individuals but that also, ironically, it is the key to an organisation's ineffectiveness.

Emotions can contribute to healthy growth if they can be harnessed appropriately, or unhealthy if they reappear unconsciously in ways which are destructive and harmful. Out of sight may be out of mind for some, but even well suppressed feelings tend to erupt into the open causing problems in relationships and in our ability to manage stressful situations and change. Fineman (1993: 15) suggests that feelings are like 'social glue', part of the 'inner wiring' of an organisation and that they 'will make or break organisational structures'.

Emotional repression in the organisation of health

Many commentators and researchers have alluded to a similar process of emotional suppression in health care, where they are viewed as dangerous and disruptive and as marginal rather than central to life at work. The medical model approach, which has been so influential in our own nursing history, tends to split off aspects of external physiological pathology from a person's own unique history, the quality of their relationships and the impact of their environment. It helps to disengage these external elements from inner emotional life. This mind–body split alienates and fragments individuals. The disturbing power of the emotions is anaesthetised and we can settle down to focus on much more manageable, compartmentalised bits that have gone wrong.

An enormous amount of both personal and organisational effort can be employed in suppressing emotions so that socially acceptable norms of relating based on composure and rationale can happen. Emotions and intuition, in a culture dominated by largely masculine values which elevate rational forms of knowing, can be seen as feminine and deviant. 'Emotional labour' in the helping and caring profession of nursing encourages benign detachment, which disguises and defends against any private feelings of pain, anxiety and distress. James (1993) explored the divisions in emotional labour with reference to disclosure about cancer and managing emotion. She refers to the 'unwritten rules' about status, gender and organisational role in shaping who says what to whom, and how their feelings are expressed:

> The mechanisms through which emotion is controlled during the disclosure of cancer are applicable to a wide range of organisations. The mechanisms may be commonly observed: the use of particular kinds of space and time: more or less public encounters; denial of the emotion; limiting the information released; formal and informal disciplinary rules; gender divided labour; and most importantly, through senior staff setting the context, routines and rituals within which other staff and clients can express their emotions.
>
> (James 1993: 114)

Davies' (1995) excellent overview of 'gender and the professional predicament in nursing' again refers to the predominant organisational logic as a masculine logic that denies the world of emotions and the need for interdependence rather than fragmentation and conflict (enhanced still more in the development of the competitive marketplace of health care). She summarises her thesis thus:

> Masculinity fears and feminises dependency. It handles vulnerability and indeed any emotional expression by handing it over to women, and

repressing and denying the need for any discussion in the rational forum of a public space.

(Davies 1995: 187)

It is why, she suggests, nurses feel so disempowered from asserting the emotional underpinning of their professional caring and the need to see this translated into organisational policy and support.

Trying to voice emotions in nursing

Many fear that if you just let a trickle of emotion out you could soon find the situation veering towards the chaotic. Workshop participants from all specialities voice these fears well:

> Her eyes filled with tears; I could tell she was desperate but the clinic was full, I had loads still to see, so I jollied her along. I feel bad about it now. But I was tired. It had been a long day. And anyway, you never know what you're letting yourself in for. The floodgates could open. Her life is in such a mess. A bit like mine really.

> All this stuff about feelings is all very well, but ITU is very pressurised. There's always relatives around and you have just got to stay in perfect control. It's really not good to get too involved. A lot of them aren't going to make it so there wouldn't be any point. If one lot of relatives start to break down then they all start. It's not so bad if they go to the visitors' room but it all gets a bit much if it happens in the unit.

> I hate going to visit him. He is always so smarmy and full of sexual innuendo. We have to do quite personal things for him. I dread going in. He makes me squirm. I just have to bottle up all my distaste and anger. There's no point. Anyway he's a friend of the Chief Exec. so I couldn't say anything anyway.

> Quite frankly we are treated like shit by the GPs, they have no idea what our role is, but we have to keep our heads down. Our manager says that if we want to keep our jobs we just have to get on with it and dance to their tune. The service contract is due for renewal soon.

Fears of catharsis, personal retribution and things generally getting out of control can mean that practitioners keep their own emotional lids on tight, and in so doing ensure that the client's needs for appropriate emotional expression are not encouraged either.

Yet many have been trying to loosen the lid in recent years; but without everyday supportive strategies and space for this, then the pace for change tends to be slow. We forget that placing emotions on the map is relatively new in health care. It is only some 20 years ago that the first nursing research linked anxiety reduction to pain relief (Hayward 1975, Boore 1978). It was then a common belief in paediatric circles that babies did not experience pain, and local analgesia was not given for many physical interventions. The therapeutic value of a more holistic approach to care based on partnership did not really gain momentum until the late 1970s and the 1980s. However, as the emotional life of clients grew to be recognised it often became a category to be ticked on a form rather than truly integrated into assessment and care. For instance, the postnatal depression scale now used extensively in community nursing can be used minimalistically or creatively depending on the skill of those using it. The Hall Report (Hall 1996) which focuses on the health of children in the community has taken ten years and three reports to shift from a more medical model approach based on childhood surveillance to the placing of children in the context of their emotional attachments and environment.

Confusing mixed messages abound. It can be disconcerting when policy documents emphasise working in partnership at the same time as tighter, more cautious procedures discourage individual practitioners' assessment and initiative. Some Trusts may become so paranoid about not missing signs of child abuse that they create policies which encourage restrictive formats for contact with whole client groups. The compartmentalisation of tasks and the increase in the use of checklists, shifts in policy which covertly affect the nurse–client relationship, can reduce individualised care and deplete confidence in the practitioner's own abilities. More recent changes in the organisation and delivery of health care and the focus on short-term measurable outcomes have led to even less emphasis on messy affective variables. The growth of feminist research in the 1970s and 1980s, with its focus on 'softer', more subjective, qualitative data, tends not to thrive in such a crude, mechanistic climate.

Although a push towards more affective methods of learning has grown in recent years, Morton-Cooper and Palmer (1993: 119) suggest that we still have a way to go:

> Given that health care is, above all, a human service, it seems reasonable if somewhat overdue, to be looking more closely at the affective domain of learning. In this way we can begin to examine our responses to emotional stressors and perhaps determine new and more acceptable ways of dealing with those that pose us with the greatest problems.
>
> Affective aspects of education could then be perceived as a legitimate subject for study, instead of being relegated to the lower ranking 'qualitative side' of educational theory. Because an approach is qualitative rather than quantitative it is sometimes accused of being too 'soft' or 'unscientific'.

Smith (1992) argues that the values of human connectedness and involvement which are so implicit in caring in nursing need to be both taught in an explicit way and underpinned organisationally. Even Benner's (1984) enormously influential overview on the philosophical roots of caring in nursing alludes to the conundrum of the 'embarrassment of caring' in an essentially masculine culture and the need to assert the centrality of its role.

This resistance to expressing and harnessing the values of emotions requires addressing in both education and practice. This is not to say that our distress should spill out all over the place all the time, but the pressure to redirect anxiety, grief, anger, stress into the deeper, non-reachable recesses of our psyche leaves us adrift from important tools for understanding ourselves and others, and from communicating with them.

Denial of feelings in nursing is particularly ironic when we all work directly or indirectly with illness, disability, threats to self-image, and fear of death and pain and all the major emotions of fear, panic, anxiety, anger, sadness and loss that accompany these states. Menzies Lyth (1988) refers to the emotional ambivalence experienced by many nurses, torn by the pull of opposite feelings: 'The work situation arouses very strong mixed feelings in the nurse; pity, compassion and love; guilt and anxiety; hatred and resentment of patients who arouse these strong feelings; envy of the care given to the patient' (Menzies Lyth 1988: 46).

Emotional well-being contributes to our overall health and satisfaction, and developing emotional skills enables our clients to utilise their own healing resources. Emotions are central and not marginal to our work and this needs to be reflected in clinical supervision. Clinical supervision has the potential for creating a space to discuss the emotional residue of our work, to identify the skills we have and those we need to develop. (See the section on emotional skills in Chapter 4.) 'Put simply, if we do not care for ourselves, we cannot care for others; if we cannot look after ourselves, we cannot look after others; if we do not respect ourselves, we cannot respect others' (Swain 1995: 29).

Implications for the relationship in clinical supervision

These undercurrents of anxiety fuelled by defensive resistance lead to a number of implications which serve to hinder the implementation or effectiveness of clinical supervision but they could provide a spur to its progress if understood and recognised. The main implications for clinical supervision we wish to highlight are the need to:

- make space for hidden feelings
- contain anxiety and conflict
- understand the subtle process of mirroring and reflecting
- recognise unconscious communication in the clinical supervision relationship and its link to clinical practice and organisational culture.

Making space for feelings in clinical supervision

This chapter seeks to redress a major imbalance in nursing education and practice which denies the power of emotions and the effect of hidden feelings in the way we relate to and communicate with others. We in no way wish to suggest that the clinical supervisor and supervisee will always be engaged in quarrying some deep dark and mysterious pit of the unknown. We are far too practical and fun-loving for that! Many aspects of clinical supervision will not involve you in unconscious processes at all.

All we are suggesting is that there needs to be more space given to explore the unconscious dynamic in education and practice, and that the clinical supervision relationship offers a time and space to incorporate this. We support and endorse Hawkins and Shohet's (1989) image of the 'wounded helper' in order that we can use rather than deny hidden but active feelings, to help both each other and our clients. To do this we need to be more aware of our own motives and needs within the helping relationship, both in direct clinical care and in clinical supervision, and acknowledge that we all have the capacity to be healed and helped by the process.

> [T]he wish to heal is basic to helpers and non-helpers alike. We have found that when we have been able to accept our own vulnerability and not defend against it, it has been a valuable experience both for us and our clients. The realisation that they could be healing us, as much as the other way around, has been very important both in their relationship with us and their growth.
>
> (Hawkins and Shohet 1989: 14)

As Maroda (1991) also suggests, this belief in the mutuality of the relationship rather than in the expert, non-disclosing authority of the role allows for some humility, true empathy and the potential for a more meaningful attachment relationship – a secure base from which to explore and try out new things.

If space is given for this then it is more likely that we can understand and so contain some of the key anxieties at work related to role and goals and identify and moderate the use of unconscious defensive ploys. Instead we can really find ways of looking after and protecting ourselves. Many of our defensive strategies grew out of a real need to protect ourselves but became as harmful as the original fears and anxieties they originally protected us from. It is more important to recognise and name what is really causing external and internal conflict and distress rather than attack or collude with it: 'Yet now more than ever, it is imperative to retain the capacity to think and act effectively under threat. If anxiety can be contained, then what needs to be talked about can be named, and some effectiveness recovered' (Mosse and Roberts 1994: 155).

Containing anxiety and conflict

In the sort of supportive, facilitating environment that clinical supervision could provide, where conflict and difference are addressed rather than avoided, the defences can be modified and the likelihood of collusion reduced. With reference to their work with community practitioners, Woodhouse and Pengelly (1991: 222) state that 'Given time, practitioners could learn from their experience of these phenomena [anxiety and defences] in an environment where conflict and anxiety were accepted and contained rather than condemned or avoided. Practitioners need such detoxifying conditions if they are to modify or appropriately relinquish defences which hinder their work.' Roberts (1994) also emphasises the need for containing space and time to encourage support and sharing and so repair the confusion created by the ideology of a caring nursing culture and the reality of the uncaring, non-nurturing climate nurses worked in.

The less we are preoccupied with defending ourselves from each other, the more energy we release and the more we expand the field of reliable and secure relationships. This can allow for more collaboration and understanding rather than merely coping or surviving in uncertainty and isolation. It involves us monitoring what the real issues are, their boundaries, possibilities and limitations. This is possible by standing back in the reflective process and helping others to do likewise in order to notice your reactions, assessing when they seem more intense than the situation may warrant, and identifying repeated patterns in the way that you relate which lead to conflict and problems. In later skills chapters we will refer to you using yourself as a 'barometer' to test out your self-reflective and awareness process within clinical supervision, and your assessment of the emotional needs of others.

Communication of hidden feelings

'It is a very remarkable thing that the unconscious of one being can react to that of another without passing through the conscious' (Freud 1915: 194). We are briefly going to explore how this can happen between individuals within the subtle but powerful silent communication of transference and counter-transference and then see how individuals may become mouthpieces for the organisation's own defences against anxiety. To acknowledge the power of unconscious communication we have to admit that we do much that is contrary to our conscious intentions, and that we are not altogether in total control of our thoughts and feelings. That is a difficult enough beginning!

We know from our experience of working with nurses that some react to such concepts as transference and counter-transference by feeling overwhelmed at their apparent complexity, and with concern that to apply this to themselves would be intrusive and 'playing counsellor or therapist'. This may reflect the shallowness of much of their previous experience of learning communication skills; teachers can also display and encourage many defensive strategies when teaching these skills. However, many nurses express relief that their experiences at last can be linked to some understandable ideas that fit and explain how they feel and what they know. Some of you may wish to return to this subsection when you have had further experience of clinical supervision or at a later stage in your development. We have found that with some skills training, nurses can learn to use 'emotional barometer' skills non-intrusively and at an appropriate level for clinical supervision. Perhaps an easier route into this is to refer to the more easily imagined mirroring and reflective process in clinical supervision.

Mirroring and reflecting in clinical supervision

Throughout this chapter and indeed the entire book, although we relate the ideas primarily to the clinical supervision relationship, this obviously does not exist in isolation. Much of what goes on between the clinical supervisor and supervisee is affected by two other main sources:

- the client: unconscious enactment in the clinical supervision relationship may reflect the dilemmas between supervisee and client
- the broader organisation: the relationship in clinical supervision is likely to mirror fundamental tensions within the organisation (Clulow 1994).

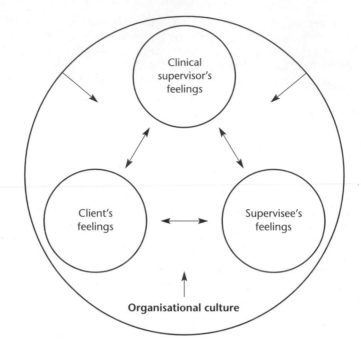

Figure 2.3 Emotional mirroring between client, supervisee, clinical supervisor within the organisational context

These interconnections and the mirroring effect between them are outlined in Figure 2.3. These mirrors can enhance and make things clearer or, like fairground mirrors, distort our image and understanding.

The link between the working alliance in clinical supervision and practice relationships has been described as the 'reflection process' (Mattinson 1975) and describes the leakage between the personal boundaries of those involved. When supervisory problems in social work were studied in a nine-year project by Mattinson it was often found that unconscious defensive interactions between the practitioner and client were being mirrored in the interaction between the clinical supervisor and supervisee. Searles's term reflection process (1955) was adopted to describe what was happening (not to be confused with the wider use of the term 'reflection' which is applied throughout the rest of this book). Woodhouse and Pengelly (1991) give a clear account of this process in the wider arena of group case discussion built on principles of clinical supervision in health care practice, where there were clear parallels between both the client's and practitioner's feelings of lack of support and isolation. The peer group then in turn had difficulty in attending both to the practitioner's clinical contact with the client and to the practitioner herself, as their own similar anxieties came into play. These involved the inner conflicts and fears inherent in anxious attachment which were reiterated by everyone, and fears about over-protection and dependency: 'She [the health visitor being supervised] conveyed a crippling sense of helplessness; of being too close and invaded by clients' (Woodhouse and Pengelly 1991: 133); this spread to her peer clinical supervision group.

Similarly the organisational defences referred to earlier can also become confused, entangled and reflected in the clinical supervision relationship. If used consciously to enable rather than disable, our understanding of the mirroring process can provide us with an effective working distance, neither so close that we are in turn immobilised, nor so out of touch that we are void of insight and unable to help.

Transference and counter-transference

Transference and counter-transference are terms used to describe how human beings use each other for unconscious purposes. Although they originated within the discipline of psychotherapy to describe aspects of the psycho-therapeutic relationship (from the viewpoint of person in therapy and the therapist respectively), they are relevant for everyone engaged in human relationships. Clearly a sophisticated in-depth understanding and applica-tion of this dynamic would be untenable and inappropriate within our own clinical discipline, but a simple description of this very common, everyday unconscious process does aid our understanding of its use within clinical supervision and in the supervisee's own clinical practice.

In clinical supervision, transference relates to the supervisee's displacement of their own internal feelings onto the supervisor. The supervisee, in their direct work with clients, in turn receives transference projections from their clients when they are in the helping role. For instance, the practitioner's sense of the client's frustration, anger or helplessness may be imported onto and felt in turn by the supervisor. Counter-transference refers to the similar process happening in reverse within the clinical supervisor (and within the supervisee in regard to their client). The clinical supervisor may not only re-experience feelings imported from their own past which the current content of the session with the supervisee or the supervisee themselves reactivate, but may also be experiencing the feelings from the clinical situation in a displaced form within the relationship with the supervisee. The task for the clinical supervisor is to try and disentangle what belongs to them and what truly belongs elsewhere, but also to use these powerful feelings as a guide to what might be happening even though it has remained unacknowledged and unsaid.

> For example, Chantal has been relating a very full and complicated account of her contact with a client with a multiplicity of health and social problems. Frank, her supervisor, suddenly realises that he has not been listening, but has instead been thinking about what shopping he needs to pick up on the way home. He has disengaged from the awfulness of her account. He realises that he has had to escape from listening to any more, and tries to put into words how disempowering this whole situation with the client must feel for Chantal, who with a frank sigh of relief admits that she just wants to run away from the whole awful mess.

Recognising the numbing effect of these feelings can not only help the practitioner know how awful in reality some situations are, which can help them not to berate themselves for not being good enough and instead recognise the boundaries of what is possible, but it can also help shift blocks and aid more creative thinking.

> Another example: Sally is feeling dismissive of her supervisee Jessica. She thinks that Jessica is hopeless in dealing with a very anxious client and feels suffocated by the 'excessive' demands being made on her clinical supervision role. Again Sally may well be picking up the desperate dependency of the client on Jessica, but Sally also recognises a very similar pattern within her own responses to demanding relationships within her personal life and personal history.

In this latter example it is easier to see how counter-transference can be a tool for good or ill. Sally may not question these old feelings which are resurfacing but choose to push them down, and distance herself from her supervisee and the problem, perhaps preferring to offer a rational solution to a 'feelings' problem. Or she could use these uncomfortable feelings to appreciate the strong ambivalent feelings for all three of them, herself, Jessica and the client, and so explore the appropriateness of the current type of supportive contact, identifying another approach which might be more anxiety-reducing and containing.

The unconscious use of roles in organisations

Bion (1967) identified the way individuals or groups could become like a 'container' for a problem that was more to do with a larger difficult dynamic within their organisation. This enables the 'problem' or 'bad bit' to be singled out but without reference to the larger underlying pathology which is denied. They remain a symptom rather than a cause. Obholzer and Roberts (1994) allude to the stress and social and political pressure within organisations which encourage this dynamic of blame. Sometimes it may lead to personal scapegoating: 'Within organisations it is often easier to ascribe a staff member's behaviour to personal problems rather than discover its link to institutional dynamics' (Halton 1994: 16), so that an individual carries something for the group that everyone finds it difficult to acknowledge and own for themselves. In clinical supervision it may be that the supervisee identifies one particular patient on the ward as a trouble-maker, always complaining and asserting their rights. In reality it may be that the standards being provided are inadequate, not because of intrinsic poor care but because the staffing levels are appalling. Fear that the patient will instigate a complaint procedure leads to staff blaming the patient. Conversely a clinical supervisor may view her newly qualified supervisee as a bit of a rebel, far too 'mouthy' and political for her own good, when she really might be saying that she and her older colleagues are too passive and frightened to rock the boat.

Non-helpful use of counter-transference

Knowledge about transference and counter-transference can also of course itself be used defensively and we need to guard against this. It can be used to great therapeutic advantage or else it can be abused. Some practitioners may choose to deny their own responsibility for monitoring their own responses, preferring to place the blame on the other person: 'Well, it's your problem not mine' or 'It's all in your mind'. They protect themselves by refusing to examine the potential reality of their contribution. As Stein says:

It is the very ordinariness and unpredictability of the transference dynamic that makes it threatening to many professionals who wish to believe that through our education, experience and will, we are in charge of our affairs – not to mention our ability to influence others. It is one matter to acknowledge that patients will transfer their own situationally inappropriate emotions and demands upon the clinician but another to accept that the clinician will do likewise to the patient.

(Stein 1985: 24)

Stein's work relates to health workers and their patients/clients but is just as relevant to the relationship in clinical supervision.

Your awareness of transference and counter-transference can be a very important tool, not only in clinical supervision but also in direct clinical care. An exploration of these everyday unconscious processes has been lacking in nursing education and we lack permission to use our vulnerabilities and the insights we can gain from them in everyday practice. Gregory (1996) alludes to this in her research on the psychosocial education of nurses: 'The professional message seems to be that to be practically competent you need to hide your vulnerability' (p. 141) and 'There seem to be many "shoulds" and "oughts" about splitting the personal from professional work under the guise of professionalism. Bringing in personal content was seen as an inferior way of working. "It could impinge" on your work' (p. 198).

Woodhouse and Pengelly (1991) found that community practitioners were similarly reluctant to acknowledge and work with the transference of anxieties from clients especially at times of stress: 'The capacity to use themselves and their knowledge wisely, think imaginatively, be curious, questioning and self observant, could desert practitioners in such situations' (Woodhouse and Pengelly 1991: 225). Hawkins and Shohet (1989) refer to the short- and long-term dangers of this. They suggest that workers who are engaged in intimate and therapeutic work with clients are:

necessarily allowing themselves to be affected by the distress, pain and fragmentation of the client and need time to become aware of how this has affected them and to deal with any reactions . . .

Not attending to these emotions soon leads to less than effective workers, who become either over identified with their clients or defended against being further affected by them. This in time leads to stress and what is commonly called burnout.

(Hawkins and Shohet 1991: 42)

Clinical supervision is a method of offering consistent and reliable backup to people who experience traumatic situations as part of their daily work with patients and clients, and suffer the strain of being employees of a politically traumatised organisation. Once nurses understand that clinical supervision is not about management interference or criticism, other hidden resistances can still come into play based on longstanding anxieties related to the emotional elements that are involved in building more responsive, supportive relationships. Yet we hope that in decades to come, this book will be redundant, that nurses will see it as an essential part of conditions of service for nurses and be shocked to hear of areas where clinical supervision is not in place.

Throughout the rest of the book we will refer to some of these hidden themes in order to see how the pitfalls and resistances can be addressed, and more skilled, effective and collaborative working alliances encouraged in clinical supervision.

Part II
Specific skills of clinical
supervision

3

The clinical supervision relationship: a working alliance

Nothing has more influence on the effectiveness of clinical supervision than the quality of the clinical supervision relationship. We acknowledge that many of the factors that make such a helping relationship work are indefinable and are affected by personal and professional histories, perceptions and reactions to each other. However, this chapter attempts to offer you some guidance in clarifying and exploring the skills you can use to create some of the conditions in which the quality of the relationship can develop, and in which hidden unconscious issues which might sabotage its success can be safely acknowledged and contained. We look at some of the elements which most concern nurses: the rights and responsibilities of the supervisee and the clinical supervisor, negotiating the clinical supervision contract and giving each other feedback. Most of the principles and frameworks in this chapter apply to one-to-one clinical supervision but we ask you to consider that the working alliance can also be between the supervisee and the members of her clinic supervision group: the group becomes the clinical supervisor and the supervisee's relationship is with the group as a whole.

At the end of the chapter we attempt to draw these strands together to ask how the clinical supervision relationship can develop into an effective working alliance. We will link back to themes explored in Chapter 2 and forward to further chapters in the book.

The quality of the clinical supervision relationship in practice

We have found that participants attending courses have reported a wide range of quality of experiences of clinical supervision as supervisees. The worst examples refer to relationships in which power is abused and the mid-range indicate some lack of understanding or skill in using clinical supervision. The most positive examples indicate commitment based on positive experiences, ability to accept the support and opportunity for development and a sense of clinical supervision being integral and essential to good clinical practice. Some comments from course participants about the quality of clinical supervision include:

> It was confidence-destroying, destructive criticism. I realise now it wasn't clinical supervision; it was just a rollicking and a badly handled rollicking at that.

> This psychologist just came in and sat in the circle and said nothing. The silence was unbearable. We ended up getting cross and he said that's what he expected. The session went on like that. Long silences till someone cracked. The woman next to me burst into tears so I held her hand and he accused me of 'rescuing'. He gave us nothing: he was only interested when people got nasty with each other, the rest of the time he looked blank. It wasn't my idea of clinical supervision so I didn't go again. It folded after three sessions, nobody would go.

> What I got was a briefing: all the information management wanted to give us via the clinical supervisor, and her collecting all the information management wanted about what was going on. There was no interest in me as a person or what I wanted to talk about. It would have been a better use of her time and ours if we'd done all that as a whole group at the staff meetings.

> I find it really difficult to think of something to talk about and sometimes she suggests a few things but they don't always interest me.

> I belong to a clinical supervision group and it's quite good, we meet once a month for an hour, but the trouble is, each person only gets to present a topic every five months, so it's not much good for burning issues, you still have to get help elsewhere. It's interesting hearing other people's problems though, you don't feel so alone. And you learn from hearing about how other people do things.

> It's OK, I've only had a few sessions. Usually I go there dreading it a bit and saying I've got nothing to talk about. But I've always ended up talking about something important and being sorry when it's time to finish. It's getting better each time.

> I'm coming up to retirement in a few years and I thought I had nothing more to learn, you know, I was just counting the days till I could retire and potter in my garden. In the last 18 months I've been having clinical supervision and quite honestly it's changed my life. I've never enjoyed my work so much as I do now. I've been on a counselling course and I now know what I'm going to do when I do retire, I'll do the full counselling training. I've even applied for a different post so that my last 18 months at work is more stimulating and so I can use counselling skills a bit more. I hope I can keep the same supervisor though. The sad thing is that it's taken so long to find out how useful clinical supervision is: it wasn't heard of when I started nursing and when it was introduced I kept putting off starting it, just couldn't imagine how helpful it could be.

What's all the fuss about? What do people mean when they can't see how they'll fit in the time? I've had clinical supervision ever since I started nursing and to me it's as important as my annual leave: if I didn't have it, I'd be less effective at work, in fact I'd be ill. The same with clinical supervision: if I hadn't had it I'd have left nursing by now, you know what it's been like in my unit. I book in my annual leave and my supervision and the rest of the work has to be fitted around that but it's not as if we've got plenty of time, we haven't. [Others in the group agreed that unit had been through a crisis and had been very short of staff.] If I didn't know I was going to have that chance to stop and think, I'd get panicky and my time management would go to pot.

Rights and responsibilities of the supervisee

Nurses attending our workshops are often very encouraged by exploring the proposition that the supervisee has specific rights: this establishes a sense of one's own power in the relationship. These also need to be set beside the responsibilities of the supervisee in order to get a balanced picture of your role as supervisee (see Table 3.1).

Your rights as a supervisee

Anxiety about clinical supervision being a hierarchical relationship in which supervisees have no rights is common. Advocating certain rights for the individual supervisee seems to set the scene for a more empowering relationship in which the supervisee can empower herself. We suggest some rights here, but encourage you to select, write in your own words and add any rights that will help you to feel strong enough to negotiate with your clinical supervisor and to use clinical supervision effectively.

As supervisee, you have the right to have some choice about who your clinical supervisor is. If you have been allocated a particular person and you do not feel sufficiently at ease with them to be able to reflect in depth on your clinical practice, then you have the right to set about arranging to have someone else. In particular, you have the right to receive clinical supervision from someone who is not your own manager or team leader: the UKCC (1996) supports this principle. Even if you work in an area where someone is employed expressly to provide clinical supervision for a number of staff, then there should be an element of choice built into the arrangement, whereby if the clinical supervision pairing is not appropriate to set up or the relationship does not work out, the supervisee can see someone else. We suggest some options in Chapter 8. We are not advocating that you have the right to have total free choice to select your clinical supervisor: this would be impractical, especially in a Trust in which the clinical supervision system is in its infancy and there are few skilled clinical supervisors available. We also support the right of the coordinator of a clinical supervision system to challenge any choices of clinical supervisor that might lead to collusive misuse of clinical supervision, such as close personal friends or relatives.

You have the right to talk about what YOU want to talk about during the clinical supervision sessions, as long as the issue ultimately has some effect on the way you do your work. You should set the major part of the agenda: the clinical supervisor may raise issues that arise from what you have said in the session or in previous ones, but the clinical supervision session is your protected time. Should you choose to talk about a personal problem outside work, you will be expected at some time to reflect on how it affects your effectiveness at work and how to maintain quality practice in spite of it: your clinical supervisor will guide you back towards linking it with work if you do not do this spontaneously. Chapter 5 suggests some differences between clinical supervision and counselling and may help clarify how you would use the two scenarios differently.

To be treated with respect as an equal partner in the working alliance is your right. This includes any decisions that affect the relationship being made with your involvement, such as, along with choice of clinical supervisor, mode of clinical supervision, whether one-to-one or group, arrangements such as times, venue, frequency of sessions. It especially means that sessions should be held in a facilitative, non-hierarchical manner which respects you as a person, irrespective of your age, gender, race or sexual orientation.

You are entitled to have anything you talk about in the clinical supervision session kept absolutely confidential, with two (possibly three) exceptions. These are: first, if you reveal any unsafe or unethical practice and you yourself are unwilling to go through the appropriate organisational procedures to deal with it; or second, you reveal any illegal activity. A third exception might be the case in Trusts where the employment contract specifies attending and making good use of clinical supervision: the clinical supervisor may have the right to contact your manager if this was not the case, though not to disclose anything you have said in clinical supervision sessions. You would have the right to know that the clinical supervisor was about to break confidentiality and to have the chance to deal with it through the normal channels yourself first. Your right to confidentiality extends to any records made of the session: you have the right to have no record made of anything personal you have talked about. We suggest in Chapter 8 that if your Trust asks for a record of the session, you provide a record showing the date and time that you attended. If you agree to include a record of topics discussed, we suggest that you write only general topic headings such as 'case review; stress management; time management; team work', etc.

You have the right to have protected time and space for the clinical supervision sessions. This means that you should have support to be released from your clinical responsibilities so you can attend. It also means that you are entitled to have the clinical supervisor give your sessions priority and stick punctually to appointments. In addition, it means that you should have an appropriate length of 'air time' in which to reflect in depth. This latter point can be a problem when clinical supervision is held in groups: we examine this difficulty in Chapter 8. Your sessions should be in private with no interruptions (except for life-or-death emergencies). You are entitled to have support to arrange cover so that you have no 'on-call' responsibilities that might lead to your being telephoned, bleeped or paged during the session.

You have the right to talk about any difficulties and vulnerable feelings, if you so wish, without being criticised or told that you are professionally incapable or that you are not coping. You are entitled to have clinical supervision with someone who can accept that your talking about these vulnerabilities in clinical supervision is a good coping strategy.

Responsibilities of the supervisee

The success of clinical supervision depends mainly on the supervisee and it can be useful to look at your responsibilities in this role. Many of the clinical supervisors attending our workshops have found that new supervisees often come expecting to hand over their problems for the clinical supervisor to solve, especially when the clinical supervisor is not seen as a peer, but is of a higher grade. This might be indicative of the dependency culture in nursing, a 'learned helplessness' resulting in expectations of the clinical supervisor as the expert problem solver.

As supervisee your primary responsibility is for the outcomes of clinical supervision, for your own development and for any actions you take in practice as a result of the sessions. It is your responsibility as a supervisee, indeed as a professional nurse, to be willing to learn and change, however experienced you are. Unfortunately, it is not uncommon for clinical supervisors attending our workshops to report having difficulties with some supervisees who give the impression of having nothing else to learn. Your clinical supervisor would have the right to challenge you if you did not take on this responsibility. It is your task to consider yourself as an equal and to empower yourself to use the clinical supervision session in the most effective way. Whilst you have the right to have the opportunities outlined earlier under 'rights', you also have the responsibility to make the most of these opportunities so that you can use the clinical supervision time effectively.

This includes taking part in negotiations about the most appropriate mode of clinical supervision, such as deciding between one-to-one or group supervision. In many Trusts, this decision is being made by working groups of representative staff who research the subject and produce guidelines for other staff. This is a participative method of introducing a clinical supervision system but its success depends on all prospective supervisees taking part in some way. This might be by letting the working group members know your viewpoint and preferences about how clinical supervision is set up, or by offering to be a working group member. When you receive guidelines about modes for clinical supervision, you need to remember that these are guidelines, not policy directives. In setting up your own clinical supervision, you have the choice about whether you follow, adapt or reject the guidelines. For instance, we worked with one group of staff who had discussed and considered the working party guidelines suggesting clinical supervision in groups. They then decided to do something different: to set up peer one-to-one supervision in their unit as this format seemed more to meet their needs.

You have the responsibility to take part in the decision about who should be the clinical supervisor for you as an individual supervisee. Even if you

Table 3.1 Rights and responsibilities of the supervisee in clinical supervision

Rights	Responsibilities
As supervisee, you have the right to:	As supervisee, you have the responsibility for:
• be treated with respect as an equal partner in the clinical supervision relationship: e.g. any decisions that affect the relationship are made with your involvement; sessions are held in a non-hierarchical setting	• asserting yourself in negotiating decisions about clinical supervision; considering yourself as an equal and empowering yourself to use the clinical supervision session in the most effective way
• some choice about the mode of clinical supervision (e.g. one-to-one or group) and who will be your clinical supervisor	• asserting yourself in negotiating the mode of clinical supervision and who will be your clinical supervisor
• set most of the agenda: to talk about what YOU want to talk about during the clinical supervision sessions, as long as the issue ultimately has some effect on the way you do your work	• preparing for clinical supervision sessions by identifying issues upon which you wish to reflect
• confidentiality, with the two exceptions of revealing unsafe or illegal practice (or third, not attending or using clinical supervision, if this is part of job contract). This includes records: you have the right to have no record made of anything personal you have talked about	• outcomes in terms of your own development and for any actions you take in practice as a result of the sessions
	• making and following through action plans that arise from your reflection during clinical supervision
• protected time for the clinical supervision sessions: support to be able to be released from your clinical responsibilities in order to attend; have the clinical supervisor give your sessions priority and stick punctually to appointments; appropriate length of 'air time'	• protecting the time for your clinical supervision by giving the appointments a high priority; turning up punctually
	• arranging cover so that you will not be 'on-call' during the clinical supervision session
• protected space for the session: in private with no interruptions; no 'on-call' responsibilities which might interrupt supervisee or clinical supervisor	• being open to challenge, not interpreting all challenges as personal attacks or discriminatory practice
• talk about any difficulties and vulnerable feelings, if you so wish, without being criticised for having these vulnerabilities	• giving feedback to the clinical supervisor about their facilitation: e.g. what is most and least helpful
	• using the time to reflect in depth on issues affecting clinical practice and avoiding non-productive conversation

have been allocated a clinical supervisor, from time to time you both need to review the relationship and establish whether your clinical supervision is with the appropriate person. If not, you need to speak up and set about arranging for someone else more appropriate to take this role.

It is your responsibility as supervisee to prepare for each clinical supervision by giving some thought to identifying issues upon which you would like to reflect. At times, this preparation will be easy since there will be burning issues on your mind. At other times, your work may be swinging along and no major events come to mind. In this case there is a danger of wasting the session time and losing an opportunity to take a wider view of your work. We offer some guidelines about preparation in Chapter 4.

Protecting the time for clinical supervision is important and it is your responsibility to give the appointments a high priority in your time management. If you have difficulty with this because of, for instance, workload, it is your responsibility to seek help from colleagues and your manager. Linked to this is your responsibility to arrange cover so that you will not be 'on-call' during the clinical supervision session.

Your learning responsibilities include being open to challenge. While clinical supervision is supposed to be fundamentally supportive, you will also be challenged on your actions, attitudes, values and knowledge and there is the possibility of important learning to be gained from this uncomfortable process. It is your responsibility to be aware of your tendencies to defend against listening to, taking some account of and learning something from being challenged. You may have a self-image of perfection or be afraid to admit to imperfection, but your responsibility is to see your way through these towards professional learning. Some defences may include interpreting all challenges as personal attacks or discriminatory practice, without examining if there is some validity about what is said. Guidelines for dealing with criticism are given later in the chapter.

Giving feedback to the clinical supervisor about their facilitation is your responsibility too. The relationship can build and become increasingly effective as you get to know each other in this special situation, and both learn more about using the time to greatest effect. Letting the clinical supervisor know what is most and least helpful is an essential part of this development. Many supervisees and clinical supervisors build in regular review sessions.

Having set up, prepared for and protected the time and space for clinical supervision, it is your responsibility to use the time to reflect in depth on issues affecting clinical practice and to avoid non-productive conversation. This can be especially difficult if you know the clinical supervisor in another role and have other mutual interests to use as red herrings.

Lastly, it is your responsibility as supervisee to make action plans after your reflection during clinical supervision, and to follow them through in practice. This links back to the first point: to be willing to learn and do things differently. These action plans may not always be about specific points of clinical procedure or management of patients or clients, they may also be about self-management, communication with colleagues or your own manager, managing other staff and so on. All these action points ultimately have a bearing on the quality of patient or client care.

Difficulties in asserting rights and taking on the responsibilities of being a supervisee

We find that lack of confidence in confidentiality as a groundrule is a common problem. This might arise from a fear of gossip. Anyone working in nursing will have experienced the extent of gossip among nurses; we have an interest in people, and their life crises and celebrations make fascinating discussion. This is not always a negative phenomenon: gossip can oil the wheels of communication in a community or organisation, keeping people in touch with each other. On the other hand, positive gossip can be spoiled by the nurse who relishes behind-the-back criticism of colleagues, and receives any personal information about them as fodder for viciousness, perhaps passing on the information to others in a distorted and damaging way. There is no foolproof method of preventing breaches of confidentiality, but some measures can help. If you emphasise how important it is to you when negotiating your clinical supervision contract, you may be able to counteract any tendency towards breaking confidentiality by impressing it on your clinical supervisor's mind. Frequent reminders and reviews of the groundrules can help, as well as having your contract visible to each of you during each clinical supervision session.

Difficulties with believing in confidentiality may be tied to mistrust of the clinical supervisor's organisational links, especially when the clinical supervisor is of a higher grade and is within the same unit or locality. Many nurses fear that revealing any personal information or difficulties in doing the job will be counted against them in developing their careers. We spoke with one group of nurses meeting to discuss the dismal career prospects of black nurses in nursing; statistics show a very small proportion of black nurses in senior positions, compared to the much higher percentage in the lower grades. Many said they felt acutely vulnerable in this respect and were adamant that they could only fully use clinical supervision if it was one-to-one and their clinical supervisor was outside their immediate management structure, i.e. from a different unit, hospital or locality within the same Trust, or even a different Trust altogether. We believe that this option should be available when setting up clinical supervision.

Fear of being judged negatively can get in the way of really using the opportunity to use the clinical supervision time effectively. This fear can be needless or realistic, based on previous experiences of poor clinical supervision. Needless fears can come from projecting your own worst critic – yourself – onto the clinical supervisor. Many nurses struggle with their inner critic who can destroy their confidence if given its head. One way of dealing with this is to tell your clinical supervisor that you tend to be over-critical of yourself and that you would like help in keeping this realistic and within bounds. Needless fears may also be based on previous experiences of receiving hurtful and incompetent criticism within nursing in settings which are totally different from clinical supervision and do not necessarily have to be replicated in clinical supervision. The structure of clinical supervision that we are advocating in this book can help to build a type of helping relationship which is new to you and these fears can be gradually diminished through the experience of taking part in it. On the other hand, realistic fears arising from previous experiences of poor clinical supervision may be more difficult to diminish. However, you can bring your learning from these experiences and ensure that they do not happen again, in setting up and following through the clinical supervision contract with another clinical supervisor.

Rights of the clinical supervisor

Whilst we find that workshop participants are more concerned with the rights of the supervisee, we feel it is important for the equality of the relationship to explore the rights of the clinical supervisor also. Taking a facilitative, empowering role such as clinical supervisor does not mean that you have to abdicate your own personal power and professional authority (see Table 3.2).

You also have the right to be treated with respect as an equal partner in the clinical supervision relationship, and not be blamed for the supervisee's own errors or failings, or for the organisation's shortcomings. If any advice or information you give is acted upon by the supervisee, those actions are still the responsibility of the supervisee.

You are entitled to break confidentiality in exceptional circumstances, which would normally have been pre-agreed with the supervisee. Suggestions about what these exceptions might be are made elsewhere in this chapter, under 'rights of the supervisee' and 'negotiating a clinical supervision contract'. You have the right to challenge any behaviour or values which the supervisee displays or talks about which give you concern about their practice, development or use of clinical supervision. Some guidance is provided in Chapter 6 on how to challenge the supervisee in a supportive way. You are also entitled to challenge any behaviour which is insulting or personally hurtful to you.

You have the right to refuse requests which make inappropriate demands on you in your role as clinical supervisor. This includes outside interference, whereby you receive requests from the supervisee's colleagues or manager to raise an issue which is their responsibility to deal with. It also includes requests from the supervisee which you consider inappropriate, such as giving practical help outside the clinical supervision sessions, providing ongoing personal counselling, or becoming a personal friend and socialising.

You are entitled to have some choice about whether or not to be the clinical supervisor of any particular supervisee. If, from knowing the supervisee previously or as you get to know her during the first session, you realise that you thoroughly dislike her or that she thoroughly dislikes you, you have the right to choose not to work with her. Having embarked on the clinical supervision relationship, you have the right to take steps to withdraw from it if there are relationship difficulties which cannot be resolved or you have difficulties in meeting the commitment.

You also have the right to set personal and professional boundaries on what issues you listen to the supervisee talking about. As a nurse and as a human being we all have limits and occasionally your boundaries may need to be asserted. There may be areas of work which are totally outside your professional expertise that you would wish to refer on to others who have the knowledge.

Table 3.2   Rights and responsibilities of the clinical supervisor

Rights	Responsibilities
As supervisor, you have the right to:	As supervisor, you have the responsibility to:
• be treated with respect as an equal partner in the clinical supervision relationship, not blamed for the supervisee's or the organisation's shortcomings • break confidentiality in exceptional pre-agreed circumstances • challenge any behaviour or values which the supervisee displays or talks about which give you concern about their practice, development or use of clinical supervision • challenge any behaviour which is insulting or personally hurtful to you • refuse requests which make inappropriate demands on you in your role as clinical supervisor, outside interference from the supervisee's colleagues or manager or inappropriate requests from the supervisee • set personal and professional boundaries on what issues you listen to the supervisee talking about • choose whether to work with a person as the clinical supervisor • take steps to withdraw from the clinical supervision relationship if you have difficulties in meeting the commitment or there are relationship difficulties which cannot be resolved	• prepare for the clinical supervision session: ensuring no interruptions; settling yourself beforehand; remembering previous sessions • be reliable, sticking to agreed appointments, time boundaries, clinical supervision contract, keep confidentiality, (except for explicitly agreed exceptions) • avoid any management or educational assessment role from being part of the clinical supervision session; to keep the session time purely within the clinical supervision contract and deal with other roles at other times • rebut inappropriate demands, e.g. outside interference from the supervisee's colleagues or manager or the supervisee trying to step over boundaries • offer 'first aid counselling' (not psychotherapy) for current burning issues but to focus on how quality professional practice can be sustained in spite of personal difficulties • encourage the supervisee to seek specialist help or advice when necessary and to have access to sources of such help • challenge any behaviour or values which the supervisee displays or talks about which give you concern about their practice, development or use of clinical supervision • ensure that you yourself have the necessary backup support, e.g. your own clinical supervision and support systems

Ursula is urgently needing guidance on child protection procedures but this is not Jan's field. She makes some suggestions about contacting experts in the Trust but has to draw the line at giving any practical guidance about it, though she is more than willing to listen to Ursula reflecting on the stress of the situation.

There may also be personal vulnerabilities which mean you are unable to listen.

George has recently returned to work after compassionate leave for a bereavement, his partner having been suddenly killed in an accident. He leaves a message to warn his supervisee Natalie, who works on a cardiac unit: 'I think you've heard what happened: well, I'm still pretty wobbly about it and I just need to say that I don't think I could manage dealing with topics directly related to bereavement: anything else, fine. If this gets in the way of any burning issues you may have, perhaps we could fix a clinical supervision session with someone else? Let me know.'

Responsibilities of the clinical supervisor

It is your responsibility to prepare for the clinical supervision session by ensuring that you will not be called or interrupted and to settle yourself before the supervisee arrives. Giving yourself space and time to remember previous sessions is important, so that you can tune in quickly to being with the supervisee as a person.

Reliability is important, such as sticking to agreed appointments and time boundaries and to the agreements made in the clinical supervision contract. You need to keep all personal information confidential, except for explicitly agreed exceptions. On the other hand, in the event of an exception arising, it is your responsibility to (1) attempt to persuade the supervisee to go through the appropriate channels herself; (2) check that this has been done; (3) and, if not, inform the supervisee that you are going to break confidentiality before doing so.

Maintaining the boundaries of clinical supervision is your responsibility. If you also have other relationships with the supervisee which involve management or educational assessment, you are expected to do this outside the clinical supervision sessions and to keep the session time purely within the clinical supervision contract. You also need to refuse requests that make inappropriate demands on you in your role as clinical supervisor, whether outside interference from the supervisee's colleagues or manager or the supervisee attempting to step over the boundaries of the working alliance.

As part of the support role in clinical supervision, it is your responsibility to offer 'first aid counselling' (not ongoing psychotherapy) for personal problems which are current burning issues for the supervisee, but eventually to focus the discussion back onto how quality professional practice can be sustained in spite of personal difficulties.

It is your responsibility to encourage the supervisee to seek specialist professional or personal help or advice when their problems are outside your field of expertise; it is also your responsibility to have access to some information about people and services available in your Trust and in the local area.

It is not only your right but your responsibility to challenge any behaviour or values which the supervisee displays or talks about which give you concern about their practice, development or use of clinical supervision.

It is your responsibility to ensure that you yourself have the necessary backup support to enable you to deal with the strains involved in being a

Table 3.3   One example of a clinical supervision agreement

As supervisee and clinical supervisor, we both agree to the following:

That the aims of our session together are to enable . . . (supervisee's name) to reflect in depth on issues affecting practice in order to develop personally and professionally towards achieving, sustaining and creatively developing a high quality of practice.

Meeting on average once per calendar month for one hour.

Protecting the time and space for . . . (supervisee's name) to reflect in depth by sticking to agreed appointments and time boundaries, being punctual, ensuring privacy and no interruptions.

Providing a record for our manager showing the dates and times of the clinical supervision sessions only. Any other notes made about the sessions during or after the sessions will be kept by . . . (supervisee's name). . . . (clinical supervisor's name) will only be given a copy when this is explicitly agreed.

Working mostly to . . . (supervisee's name)'s agenda.

Working in the spirit of learning about how to use clinical supervision, both of us being open to feedback about how we handle the clinical supervision sessions.

Challenge any breach of this clinical supervision agreement which the other does not already acknowledge or does not take seriously enough.

As supervisee I agree to:

Prepare for the sessions and be responsible for having an agenda.

Take responsibility for making effective use of the time, for the outcomes and any actions I take as a result of clinical supervision.

Be willing to learn and change and to be open to receiving support and challenge to help me do so.

As clinical supervisor, I agree to:

Keep all personal information you reveal in the clinical supervision sessions confidential, except for these exceptions: (A) you reveal any unsafe, unethical or illegal practice and you yourself are unwilling to go through the appropriate organisational procedures to deal with it; (B) you repeatedly don't turn up for sessions or do not use the time constructively. In the event of an exception arising, I will (1) attempt to persuade and support you to deal with the issue directly yourself through the appropriate channels; (2) check that this has been done; and (3) if not, only reveal the information as a last resort after informing you that I am going to do so.

Not allow any management supervision or educational assessment role to be part of the clinical supervision session.

Offer you support, catalytic help, supportive challenge and information or advice to enable you to reflect in depth on issues affecting your clinical practice.

Use my own clinical supervision to support and develop my own abilities in working with you, without breaking confidentiality.

Signed _____ supervisee
       _____ clinical supervisor

clinical supervisor. This includes having your own clinical supervision and developing and using your own support systems.

Negotiating a clinical supervision contract

Every relationship between people is based on their expectations of each other. The relationship goes well when expectations are met and goes badly when they are not, leading to disappointment, disruption, a sense of betrayal and even breakdown of the relationship in extreme cases. These expectations may be explicit, such as those laid out in an employment contract, but the majority are implicit. Open discussion of expectations can help establish and maintain a relationship and go towards healing one that is going wrong. In many informal relationships it would be stilted and unnatural to negotiate a contract at the outset ('I'd like to be your friend and draw up a friendship contract'!). However, clinical supervision is a formalised type of professional support, in which the people involved meet fairly infrequently; therefore it is important that the supervisee and clinical supervisor make an agreement about how they work together in clinical supervision (see Table 3.3). This helps to clarify expectations of each other, gives you both the same view of where you are going, builds trust when the supervisee and clinical supervisor come to see the agreement enacted in practice and provides a common language for talking about and reviewing the working relationship. We suggest four steps in negotiating such a contract.

1 Both of you talk about what you want from each other in clinical supervision, your understanding of the aims of clinical supervision, your hopes and fears, why you chose each other and so on. Notes you take from this discussion can form the beginning of a draft agreement.
2 You write out a draft agreement and agree which points to include and how to word them so that both your understandings are reflected. You could consult the draft given in Table 3.3 or any guidelines produced in your Trust and incorporate any points that are important to you.
3 Your agreement is signed, with both having a copy: preferably the supervisee keeping the original, and the clinical supervisor keeping the duplicate.
4 The contract is reviewed at regular intervals and if necessary revised.

The beginning of the process is illustrated by the following example.

Liam and Sandra spend the first clinical supervision session together talking through and agreeing the contract. Liam has had clinical supervision before in a previous job, and Sandra is a clinical supervisor for the first time, and has only recently begun to receive clinical supervision herself. They begin by Sandra asking: 'Shall we start with our hopes and fears? What do you hope to get from clinical supervision with me, Liam?' Liam: 'Well, I got a lot out of it with my last clinical supervisor, not particularly the first one I had, but the second one worked out well, so I hope I'll get the same.' Sandra: 'And that was . . . ?' Liam: 'Richard helped a lot, listened, was a sort of sounding board, and when he criticised, it was constructive criticism, it was all right. And especially with him, he was there: he turned up on time and never cancelled sessions, except once when his mother died, but otherwise I knew I could count on him.' Sandra: 'OK if I write these down? So, you'd like from me: listening, sounding board, constructive criticism, punctuality, reliability – not cancelling sessions. Anything else come to mind?' Liam: 'Thinking about fears: what I dread is having the same set-up as the first time. We'd fix dates and she hardly ever kept to them, I know she was off sick quite a bit and she had to keep going to emergency management meetings because her unit was going to be closed at one stage, but when we did manage to have a session she was usually late. It was a waste of time.' Sandra: 'I can't forecast being sick and having closures but suppose something like that happened and I just couldn't stick to appointments, would it be better if we suggested another clinical supervisor is found for you?' Liam: 'Yes, that's what happened eventually, I had to find someone else and it turned out OK then, but I'd wasted a lot of time and I didn't think much of clinical supervision for a while.' Sandra: 'So we'll keep our fingers crossed, but do something about it quickly if it looks as if it's going that way. Actually, that ties in with what I wrote down about wanting from you: I'd hope you would turn up when we said and be on time, because I can't really run late with sessions. So we're both concerned about punctuality. Another one of mine is feedback: as you know, I have less experience of clinical supervision than you do and I'd like feedback about what is and isn't helpful, so I can learn. What do think about those?' After some discussion Sandra suggests: 'There's some more things on the groundrules put forward by the working group, what do you think of these?' They go on to draw up their agreement, emphasising their special concerns and prompted by the suggestions shown in their local guidelines.

Pitfalls in negotiating a clinical supervision contract

One common pitfall for people new to clinical supervision is blindly adopting a pre-written contract, such as that in Table 3.3 or those produced in some Trusts by working parties. This can result in lack of ownership of the agreement: the individual supervisee and clinical supervisor not fully understanding what each other means by each point and feeling less committed to the agreement than would be the case if they devised it together. To avoid this, we suggest you have the initial discussion as suggested earlier, and draft some of your own groundrules together as a result of this discussion, before you refer to any other guidelines.

Sometimes nurses make heavy weather out of writing such contracts, expecting that this written agreement has to be beautifully presented, typed and written in complicated language as if it were some legal document or Trust policy document. Some try to standardise such agreements, spending precious time in liaising across units, localities or throughout the Trust. However, we maintain that the agreement needs to be a record of what you as individual people understood and agreed between you and does not have to be comprehensible or seen by anyone else or standardised along with other clinical supervision pairs or groups.

Another pitfall is to make the contract, then file it away without referring to it again. This can result in either or both of you forgetting about the agreement and being more likely to break it. It may result in a growing suspicion in the supervisee that the agreement was just a paper exercise and had no lasting meaning. Suggestions made earlier about using the agreement as part of regular reviews and having it on display during sessions can help keep the agreement alive.

Not preparing a written contract at all may be tempting to nurses who have had some experience in clinical supervision or who know each other already. This can lead eventually to misunderstandings of each other and some unnecessary conflicts. The process of working together on a written agreement is an important step in establishing the structure, boundaries and mutual understanding necessary for such a specific type of helping relationship as clinical supervision.

Writing points such as 'trust' and 'respect' into groundrules is too vague to be particularly helpful. These essential elements of an effective working alliance are the hoped-for outcomes of contract setting, but in agreeing the contract, it is more helpful to be specific about the kinds of behaviour that would help build trust and would demonstrate respect.

Discussing the working alliance

We recommend that clinical supervisor and supervisee together review the way the clinical supervision relationship is developing. This is especially important in the first year and if either or both are new to clinical supervision, in order to assist mutual learning. Longer established clinical supervision relationships can be much enhanced by reviews, preventing unhelpful habits becoming established or clearing up possible points for resentment that otherwise might gradually sour the relationship. These reviews can be structured or ad hoc.

A structured review can be built into the clinical supervision contract as an agreement to review the relationship at regular intervals. The format of the review could proceed as follows:

1 *Review of contract*: the supervisee states which of the groundrules in the contract she feels that she has upheld and which she has not. The clinical supervisor gives feedback to the supervisee about this, sharing any concerns and appreciations. The clinical supervisor then states which of the groundrules she has upheld and which she has not, and the supervisee gives feedback. Any necessary revision to the contract is made in the light of this sharing.

2 *Review of the clinical supervisor's facilitation*: the clinical supervisor gives a brief self-assessment under these two headings: 'How I think I have been most effective as a clinical supervisor; what I would like to do differently in the future'. The supervisee responds to this self-assessment, or gives feedback along the same lines: 'What I appreciate most about the way you

carry out your role as my clinical supervisor; what I would like different in the future from you'. One important principle is that the supervisee comments only on behaviours, not the personality of the clinical supervisor. A second is that there should be a balance between positives and negatives, otherwise the review is likely to be experienced by the clinical supervisor as an attack or as too cosy.

3 *Review of the supervisee's use of the clinical supervision sessions*: the supervisee first makes a self-assessment, covering the following two points: 'Some ways in which I think I'm making effective use of the clinical supervision sessions' and 'Some ways in which I could make more effective use of the sessions in the future'. The clinical supervisor reacts to the self-assessment or shares points under similar headings, again with comments only on behaviours, not personality, giving a balance between positives and 'do differentlies'.

Liam and Sandra are having a review of their first three clinical supervision sessions. Liam: 'I feel that I have kept to the groundrules, though I think I could have probably given you some more feedback on the spot, as I'd agreed to do.' Sandra agreed but reminded him of one occasion when he stopped her when she was giving some unwanted advice: she found it helpful to be reminded to check if advice is wanted. She also suggested that he need not be so wary in telling her about difficulties with a particular colleague, that she would definitely keep it confidential. Sandra then assessed herself as having met the groundrules as agreed but wanted to clarify the confidentiality groundrule a bit more. When they made the contract, she had not specified that she herself would be using her clinical supervision to reflect on her role as clinical supervisor, and whilst this meant disclosing a little of the content of the sessions, she wanted to assure him that this was done without identifying him or anyone he talked about and was more focused on her own issues and development. Liam: 'That's OK with me but I'm glad we got it clear: I was wondering about it. What I'd like to say is that I've really appreciated you being reliable about the appointments and being a sounding board, plus you've given me some good ideas, especially that problem last time. The "do differently" is what we said earlier, perhaps wait until I'm ready before you give advice.'

Ad hoc feedback can be given at any time. As supervisee, you may feel that a certain part of a clinical supervision session has been especially helpful: you could say so at the time and specify exactly what the clinical supervisor did that was so helpful. You may be struggling with an issue and finding that the clinical supervisor's interventions are not useful to you: saying so at the time gives the clinical supervisor a chance to adapt the approach so that it is more effective. As clinical supervisor, you may be impressed with some aspects of the way the supervisee works in clinical supervision and it can be very encouraging to say this at the time. You may notice some way in which the supervisee is hampering herself, not making best use of the time: it can be facilitative to share this at the time.

More guidance on giving encouragement is given in Chapter 5, and on challenging in Chapter 6. Whilst these pointers are focused on the clinical supervisor's facilitative role, the supervisee may also find the guidelines helpful when considering giving feedback to the clinical supervisor.

Dealing with criticism in clinical supervision

We find that most nurses receiving training in supervisee skills request some help with learning how to deal with criticism. Often there is some anxiety behind the request, based on the misapprehension that clinical supervision will involve a lot of criticism. On the contrary, the major part of the work of the clinical supervisor is support and catalytic help (see Chapter 5). However, at times, the clinical supervisor will challenge (i.e. constructively criticise) the supervisee to increase awareness of the part she herself might play in some of the problems under discussion.

Your clinical supervisor's intention and manner should be supportive and aimed at enabling you to learn and develop. However carefully and skilfully the clinical supervisor makes these challenges, it is likely that, as supervisee, you will feel some discomfort. Most people do when criticised, however constructively it is done. Similarly, participants on clinical supervisor training courses often request help with dealing with criticism from supervisees who are encouraged to give feedback about what is helpful and not helpful. Clinical supervisors realise that they are not going to be perfect in their clinical supervisor role and also feel nervous about the prospect of being challenged.

Whether as supervisee or clinical supervisor, your emotional reaction to the experience of being challenged is likely to be affected by your past experiences. Most nurses have been on the receiving end of criticism which has been badly given, unjust, badly timed or humiliating, whether during their working time or elsewhere. Fear of being demolished by destructive criticism leads to many of the defensive practices explored in Chapter 2. In Clulow's (1994) study of supervisory relationships, he found there was a great deal of anxiety on both sides about their own competence and whether it was safe for either of them to reveal any lack of confidence however transitory; there was a deep fear that disclosure would be criticised. Even the most constructive, well-timed, supportive criticism can make you feel terrible if you have been humiliated a lot in the past. As a result, it can be easy to over-react to even the most skilled, sensitive clinical supervisor or perhaps to under-react to someone who is mistaken or being unjust. The guidelines offered here suggest a few ways of dealing with criticism which might help you to cope with the discomfort and to learn something from the situation.

Consider the steps shown in Figure 3.1. First of all, when you are challenged, listen and take time to collect yourself and think about what has been said. If your clinical supervisor does not spontaneously give you space to reflect, then ask for it.

Carol describes how an elderly patient was discharged home too early because the bed was needed for an emergency admission, and subsequently had to be readmitted after a serious fall. She describes

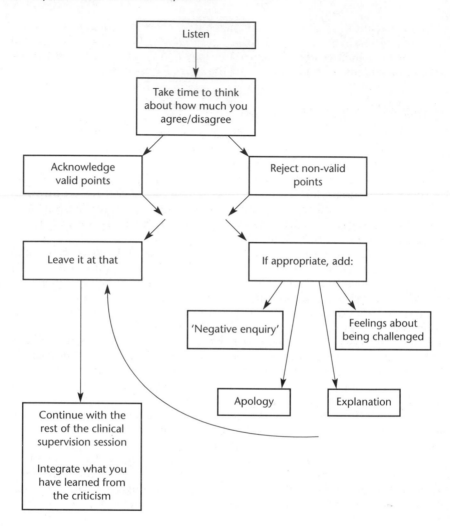

Figure 3.1 Steps in dealing with criticism

trying to stand up to the consultant but was rebuffed by a rude response. David, her clinical supervisor: 'It sounds as if you gave up at the first hurdle and didn't try to persist to show how important your viewpoint was'. Carol: 'Well, I need to think about that', and she takes a few moments to cast her mind back over the situation.

Next, decide how much truth there is in it, if any. Categorise the criticism as either 'I totally agree', or 'I totally disagree', or 'I partially agree (i.e. 'I agree with part of it, but disagree with the rest').

Malcolm is a professional support worker whose role includes providing clinical supervision along with other development tasks within that sector of the Trust. His Trust has instigated a new training initiative and Malcolm is under pressure to enlist participants. During Nora's clinical supervision session with him, he gives quite a lot of information about this initiative and tries to persuade Nora to sign up for it. Nora says: 'Malcolm, look, this is quite interesting but this is not meeting my needs at the moment. I'm really worried about the problem I tried to discuss with you but this training initiative is your agenda. I thought this was supposed to be my time.' He realises straight away that she is right.

If you think the challenge is accurate, then try to accept the valid criticism, however embarrassing it feels to admit to it. State that you agree with the criticism: a plain, direct, honest answer deals positively with the criticism and helps you to let it sink in and to learn from it. Accept valid criticism without defensive justifications, excuses, passing the buck and so on. If you talk or sidle your way out of it, you are likely to learn less from it.

Carol continues: 'Yes you're right, I didn't keep at it.' ﹐

Malcolm responds to Nora: 'That's quite true, I made a mistake pushing my agenda so much.'

If you think the criticism is inaccurate, then state that you disagree with the criticism and contradict it with a positive statement about yourself. You need to reject criticism with which you disagree, without retaliating. The other person is unlikely to put you down for the sake of it, they may just be mistaken. So, just respond by saying that you disagree and contradict the critical statement with a positive statement about yourself.

Veronica is telling her clinical supervisor Margaret about a complicated situation in which two of her staff nurses were in conflict with each other and refusing to cooperate. She had asked a particular third year student nurse to go and work with them and had briefed her about the conflict. Margaret: 'I wonder if you were a bit rash to delegate to a student the job of sorting out the staff nurses?' Veronica: 'Well, actually, I disagree. I think I made a very good choice.'

If the challenge has some truth in it but is overstated or slightly off beam, then specify exactly what you agree with and what exactly you disagree with.

Patrick, Annette's clinical supervisor: 'I'm concerned that you're always late for our sessions together.' Annette: 'Granted I was today and a bit last time but I disagree with your saying "always" because I've been punctual every other time.'

At times, it is sufficient to show agreement or disagreement and leave it at that. You can then go on with the clinical supervision session and build into it what you have learned from the criticism. As supervisee, you might be able to use it in your reflection on the issue that you have brought to clinical supervision. As clinical supervisor, you might be able to use what you learned by adapting your approach during the rest of the session.

At other times, additional responses to criticism may be appropriate, though beware of saying too much out of anxiety. 'Negative inquiry' involves asking questions to elicit more useful details from a clinical supervisor who is challenging you or who you think might be feeling critical of you, but not expressing it. The word 'negative' may seem confusing here, but this is the term you will find used in the classic books about assertive communication, such as Dickson (1982). It is actually 'positive' in the sense that you are enabling your critic to give constructive rather than destructive criticism. This is based on the belief that constructive criticism is helpful and, applied to clinical supervision, that the supervisee wants to learn from being usefully challenged.

Situations in which 'negative inquiry' may be helpful include: when you disagree with the other person when they have not given you enough information so that you can understand what they mean; when you think the other person is concerned or critical but has not expressed it; when they have used a generalisation such as 'always' or have commented on your personality rather than your behaviour or manner.

'Negative inquiry' can help you to find out exactly what actions you've done or what type of approach has bothered them. It can also help you to discover the emotional effects of your actions. So, you can use this knowledge by taking it into account next time you act. Alternatively it can open up a useful discussion about viewpoints and values.

'What was it that concerned you about my being late?' This went on to become a useful discussion about Annette's commitment to clinical supervision.

Veronica asks: 'What made you think that it was a bad decision?'

Giving a reason may be appropriate, especially if it is about the clinical supervision session itself or about your professional practice. Explaining what happened may clear up misunderstandings, but beware of using reasons as excuses or justifications to deflect a useful challenge.

Annette explains that today and last time, there were crises on the ward just before she was due to leave for the clinical supervision session and she felt that she had to complete what she was doing rather than try to hand over to someone. This led to a discussion about the timing of clinical supervision sessions and they agreed in future to hold the sessions at a different time of day, when Annette was less likely to get embroiled.

In Carol's case, there was no need to explain why she found it difficult to persist, as she had already described the difficulties of the situation and a repetition would just have been a defensive justification. Instead, they went on to explore how Carol could persist with getting her points across with this particular consultant the next time she disagreed with him.

It seemed appropriate for Veronica to explain: 'The student is a mature student, older than both the staff nurses, she used to be a school teacher. She's really good at laughing off this type of nonsense and as it turned out, she managed to get them both laughing about how stupid it was. That team did really good work that shift.'

The person making the challenge may be entitled to an apology for something that affects her, and it might help to say what you are prepared to do about it in future.

Annette: 'I really am sorry I kept you waiting and made you wonder if I'm not bothered about clinical supervision. Now we've changed the times I'll move heaven and earth to get here on time.' Malcolm adds: 'I'm sorry. Let's go back to what you were saying about the problem with so-and-so.'

There may be a place for sharing how you feel emotionally about being challenged or about the way the other person has challenged you.

Annette: 'I feel disappointed that you questioned my commitment to clinical supervision. I've put a lot into getting here and working with you and I've done a lot to get some colleagues thinking more positively about it too.'

These methods and examples may sound uncomfortable and some may fear that such methods would damage the working alliance. We maintain that it is not appropriate to strive to feel comfortable all the time in clinical supervision: getting things into the open, surfacing hidden tensions and clearing up misunderstandings are essential for an effective working alliance.

Pitfalls in dealing with criticism

The almost inevitable discomfort of being on the receiving end of a challenge can lead to non-assertive approaches; that is, being aggressive, manipulative or submissive (see Table 3.4). An aggressive approach to dealing with criticism includes various ways of attacking in retaliation. These might include dragging up some real or imagined mistake or fault on the part of the person doing the criticising, and using it to attack them. For instance, if Annette had retaliated with 'What about you? You can talk! You were late for the very first meeting', then the discussion might have degenerated into an argument, instead of leading to some useful discussion. Retaliation might be in the form of automatically accusing the person of gender or racial discrimination, without first considering if there might be some truth in the criticism. Other aggressive responses include not listening, interrupting a lot, walking out of the session, blaming the person doing the criticising or refusing to rectify a mistake out of spite.

A submissive approach to dealing with criticism involves not setting limits or not standing up for yourself. You might be allowing people to get away with unjust or badly given criticism. It would be submissive to allow the other person to label your personality without asking them to be more specific

Table 3.4   Pitfalls in dealing with criticism

Aggressive approach
   Retaliating by pointing out the faults of the person doing the criticising
   Retaliating by automatically accusing the person of discriminatory practice
   Not listening, interrupting a lot
   Walking out of the session
   Refusing to rectify a mistake out of spite

Submissive approach
   Allowing people to get away with unjust or badly given criticism
   Allowing the other person to label your personality without asking them to be
      more specific about your actions
   Accepting criticism second-hand instead of going to face the critic in person
   Being over-apologetic
   Absorbing all criticism, whether valid or not, and using it to feed a negative
      self-image

Indirect approach
   Blaming someone else
   Trying to talk the other person into changing their mind
   Throwing in red herrings
   'Poor me': trying to get the person doing the criticising to feel sorry for you
   Criticising the manner of the criticism, whilst ignoring valid content
   Insincerely appearing to agree with valid criticism

---

about which of your actions they are concerned. Submission might include
accepting criticism second-hand instead of going to face the critic in person.
Accepting too much of the criticism is submissive; perhaps being over-
apologetic or, at the extreme, absorbing all criticism (whether valid or not)
and using it to feed a negative self-image. For instance, Veronica would have
been submissive if she had responded to the inaccurate criticism with 'OK,
yes, I've been told I'm hopeless at delegating, I always have been.'

   The manipulative or indirect approach to dealing with criticism involves
deflecting the criticism in a manner which is not explicitly aggressive. Some
ways of talking your way out of facing up to the criticism might include blaming someone else, trying to talk the other person into changing their mind
or throwing in red herrings. The indirect approach might include trying to
get the person doing the criticising to feel sorry for you or criticising the way
they gave the criticism, while refusing to acknowledge any validity in the
content of what was said. Lastly, it might involve appearing to agree with
valid criticism, but just doing it to smooth things over. Annette would have
been indirect if she had given excuses at length, blaming a colleague for
incompetence and management for not providing cover (without being asked)
and so on.

   It is the aggressive, submissive and indirect approaches which can cause
lasting damage to a working relationship, rather than the assertive approaches
suggested earlier.

   In response to the anxieties many nurses have expressed to us about dealing with criticism, we have given over quite a lot of space in this chapter to

offering practical guidelines on this but we wish to emphasise that this forms a very small part of an effective clinical supervision relationship. You might ask, 'How do you know if the relationship is effective?'

Features of an effective clinical supervision relationship

Imagine that you could be a fly on the wall of some clinical supervision sessions which are going well, and consider what your criteria would be for describing a clinical supervision relationship as effective. Identifying your criteria might be a useful joint exercise to add to the review structure suggested earlier in this chapter, with some exploration of what issues are emerging between you which are blocking the potential effectiveness of your working alliance. We have been lucky enough to observe many actual and practice clinical supervision sessions during consultancy work and training sessions, and will try to paint a picture here of an effective working alliance.

Seeing the relationship in action over a number of sessions, we note that the atmosphere is fundamentally one of support and advocacy for the supervisee, with the focus on the supervisee leading the session with their agenda. The clinical supervisor shows a genuine interest in the supervisee as a person, and in the patients/clients and the context in which the supervisee works: it is almost as if some of the significant people with whom the supervisee works are in the room. There is a fairly relaxed beginning to each session, with short periods of general chat and there has obviously been some good communication about expectations and about the process of working together because they have a sort of shorthand language about what is wanted from the session and about how they will proceed.

In spite of the relaxed beginning there is still a slight air of formality with a certain amount of tension as complex issues are grappled with and, at times, the supervisee is obviously feeling challenged to examine their awareness of self, own behaviour, strengths, weaknesses, feelings and values. From time to time, there is some attempt to clarify what type of help the supervisee requires: the supervisee pauses and asks for some specific type of help from the clinical supervisor, such as helping to find a direction through the complexity, or giving some advice or information. The clinical supervisor checks occasionally if the supervisee is getting what is wanted. At times, there is some humour, expressing enjoyment at achieving something or a sense of the ridiculous, or as a tension release, but it is not at anyone's expense, and not diverting from the task. The energy seems to go in waves, settling at the beginning of the session, winding down towards the end and in between punctuated by periods of intense work with pauses to recap and complete each phase or topic.

However, not everything goes smoothly. There are times when the supervisee seems to be in a complete muddle and times when either or both the supervisee and clinical supervisor seem at a loss to know how to sort it out, perhaps one or other or both of them saying so. Eventually they both come out of the confusion with the supervisee developing some new insights about the complex issue under discussion. Occasionally there is disagreement or resentment between them, which causes a little tension but they explore it, accept it, recover and move on. There is an openness in the relationship: for instance, occasionally, there are disclosures of some uncertainties or personal vulnerabilities in their respective roles, either or both confessing to finding the process difficult. The supervisee has enough trust in themselves and the clinical supervisor to reveal some of the personal difficulties and mistakes that they experience in whatever aspects of their work they are addressing in the sessions.

There is a sense of mutual enquiry. The supervisee brings complicated issues which have no single answers and they explore them together. The clinical supervisor is obviously equally curious as to where the discussion will lead them and how things will turn out in reality. There is an atmosphere of joint endeavour: supervisee and clinical supervisor seem tuned into and paying attention to one another. The work that is done in the sessions involves the supervisee in in-depth reflection on practice situations and issues affecting that practice. The beginning of each session usually includes a report by the supervisee of how s/he has put into practice the learning from the last session. Each session usually ends with some clarity on the supervisee's part about what has been achieved during the clinical supervision session and how it will be put into practice.

This chapter has offered some practical guidelines for clarifying rights and responsibilities, negotiating the clinical supervision contract, and reviewing the relationship with the intention of equipping you to develop an appropriate symmetry of power in the relationship and the building of a secure psychological base for the supervisee within the organisation. Linking back to the structural discrimination issues and blocking factors highlighted in Chapter 2, we urge you to be alert to and honest about your own prejudices, negative attitudes towards each other, any stereotypes that the other may trigger for you and your fears about clinical supervision itself; and that you seek to minimise their destructive influences on the clinical supervision relationship. Whilst the work in this chapter has aimed towards providing appropriate boundaries, and taking responsibility for the quality of the relationship, other conditions for developing effective working alliances depend on committed management sponsorship, choice of clinical supervisor, choice of delivery framework, allocation of appropriate amount of protected time, skills training and continuity: these are explored in Chapter 8.

The next four chapters focus in turn on the reflective skills of the supervisee, the enabling skills of the clinical supervisor and the skills of group clinical supervision. Whilst we have had to separate these out of necessity, we would like you consider all within the context of the clinical supervision relationship. This working alliance between supervisee and clinical supervisor aims towards providing a secure psychological base for the supervisee within which to feel safe enough to grasp the nettle of accepting support for vulnerabilities, considering challenges to actions, values and attitudes, and reflecting in depth on their own clinical practice and their own part in it.

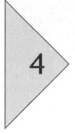

4 Reflective skills of the supervisee

This chapter aims to provide some practical frameworks to help you with the reflective process of clinical supervision, with the long term aim of enabling you to integrate this process into your everyday practice. It highlights the need for balance between analytical thinking skills and those of emotional understanding and expression. Both these areas of skills are needed to foster creative reflective practice. Clinical supervision can provide a space to try out these skills and in so doing allow the supervisee, with the help of the clinical supervisor or members of a clinical supervision group, to identify the skills they already have proficiency in and those that are less easily available to them.

How you as supervisee use clinical supervision time to think about, select from, describe, be critical about, disclose and so on, will also in part reflect the skills you have honed and developed in your personal life. Earlier attachment and educational histories may affect the range of thinking and emotional skills immediately at your disposal. The frameworks offered in this chapter must be seen in the context of the clinical supervision relationship: time must be allowed for enough feelings of trust and self-confidence to develop before the frameworks can be used effectively as part of the working alliance. Not all of the this chapter will be relevant to every reader, but some of the guidelines may enable you to identify some of the gaps in your skills and reflect on them with reference to the blocks and attachment implications explored in Chapter 2.

In this chapter we also wish to distinguish between reflection *on* practice and reflection *in* practice. This distinction relates to Fish *et al.*'s (1989) terms 'learning *from* practice' and 'learning *through* practice'. Learning from practice suggests that there is an ideal way to practice, sanctioned by theory and the 'way it is done around here'. Learning through practice suggests more of a dynamic process 'through which to learn something wider and of more significance' (Fish *et al.* 1989: 32). This more sophisticated absorption and integration of a range of skills allows for on-the-spot processing, reflection, prioritising and action as appropriate, so that you both 'do' and refine practice at the same time. In clinical supervision, a similar developmental process can happen, moving from being in supervision with a clinical supervisor or group where reflection *on* practice can take place, to developing your own 'internal supervisor'. This 'internal supervisor' is the part of you that internalises the composite mixture of skills developed with the help of the clinical supervisor, to use 'on the job' as reflection *in* practice. Implicit in 'internal supervision' is the processing of the relationship and communication elements of your work with the client, as well as the more technical aspects of clinical practice.

The chapter looks at:

- preparing for a supervision session by focusing on some topics for reflection and beginning the reflective process
- some practical methods of intuitive and step-by-step reflection
- developing your 'internal supervisor'.

In your everyday work you make thousands of decisions and solve hundreds of problems, often without needing to stop and think too much about doing so. The work involved in nursing requires you to be alert to the people around you, constantly observing and assessing needs and resources, and to make decisions and act quickly to get practical tasks done. Stopping to think about a complicated issue or an overview of some aspect of your work, and focusing on your own part in it, requires a different mind set: the mental and emotional skills of introspection. We find that nurses often have difficulty making that transition between external busy-ness and introspection and that this difficulty can lie at the heart of problems in being able to make the best use of clinical supervision. Dartington (1994: 101) suggests that:

> Contemporary nursing has been dogged by a negative expectation that nurses should not think, that is: to engage in a process of reflection about one's work, its efficacy and significance, registering what one observes of the patient's emotional state, the capacity to be informed by one's imagination and intuition, the opportunity to criticise constructively and to influence the working environment. It is an effort of will to make space for reflection in a working life dominated by necessity, tradition and obedience.

The experienced practitioners attending our clinical supervision courses are usually action-oriented in day-to-day work and often express or display this difficulty in switching from paying attention to external events going on around to paying attention to thoughts and feelings going on within. These experienced nurses find that the range of frameworks we offer in this chapter is useful for selecting appropriate methods of making the transition. More recently trained nurses who have had reflective skills building as an intrinsic part of their basic nurse training also find some value in revisiting reflective frameworks to develop their skills in wider and deeper directions (see Figure 4.1).

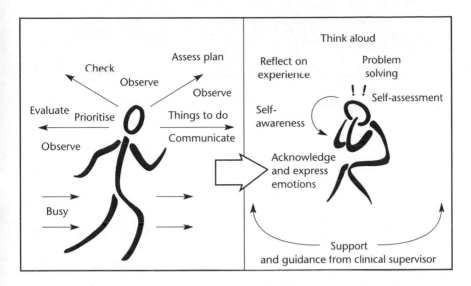

Figure 4.1 Transition between action-oriented work to reflection on practice

Preparing for a clinical supervision session

As supervisee, it is important that you give some thought to your agenda for the clinical supervision session, and to make a start at reflecting on those topics. Preparation will help you to make the transition from action-oriented work to in-depth reflection during clinical supervision (see Figure 4.1). The opportunity for you to be empowered to use the session as your time for reflection will be lost if you are unable to initiate the work. Sometimes the choice of topic will be straightforward since you may have a burning issue on your mind that you have already tried to think through on your own and for which you have a pressing need for support and guidance. At other times, you may find it difficult to think of something to bring to the session.

Figure 4.2 and the following suggestions may help you plan your agenda. To find a relevant issue for reflection, you could scan through each of the four main areas shown in Figure 4.2. Consider your care of a specific patient or client, including establishing the relationship, care assessment and planning, technical nursing procedures, communication about care plans and progress, emotional support, health education, work with their family or carers, delegation to and monitoring of other nurses, evaluation of care, preparation for transfer and finishing the relationship. Alternatively, you could focus on one area of responsibility in your role or your caseload, such as caseload management, team work, time management, management of junior staff, training of staff and students, specialities within your role and so on.

Your need may be more to explore some of the stresses or pressures arising from the job. You could consider the stresses that arise from the nature of

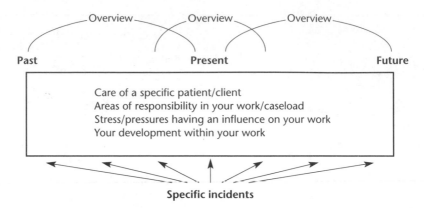

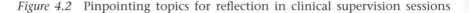

Figure 4.2   Pinpointing topics for reflection in clinical supervision sessions

your work with patients, clients or their families, from communicating with other nurses and professionals or from working within the organisation. Alternatively, you could look at stresses from elsewhere in your life which have an influence on your work: it can be relevant to look at personal stresses provided you relate your reflection to finding ways of maintaining your standards at work in spite of those difficulties. Lastly, you could consider your development as a person and as a professional within your work. You could ask yourself what personal qualities and professional expertise are being utilised and developed within your work or those which you would like to develop more in the future.

You could tackle any one of these from two perspectives: taking an overview or focusing on specific incidents. You could think in terms of scanning a particular span of time, choosing perhaps to review the past or the recent past/present/near future, or to consider the long-term future. Alternatively, you could focus on specific complicated events, whether in the past, recently, in the present or anticipated in the near or long-term future.

If considering these general areas does not fully enable you to pinpoint your agenda, the following prompts may help you to focus.

Your care of a particular patient or client: specific incidents

Think back over your recent work with this client or patient and pick out something that went well or not so well. Pinpoint anything about working with this patient or client that had an impact on you, whether you were concerned, upset or pleased about it. Alternatively, scan further back in your time working with this client or patient and notice any events that pop into your mind, even though they are long past. Notice especially those which have an emotional charge to them, for instance those situations in which you felt helpless, embarrassed, sad, angry, pleased with yourself, happy, etc. You could scan back using any of these emotions as a theme, for instance: 'Times when I've felt helpless working with X'. You could try looking to the future: cast your mind forward to any complex situations that the patient or client will have to deal with with your help, in the near future. Anticipate any major event which is likely to happen to the patient or client in years to come, whether you will be involved in the care or not. Consider how you and the patient or client can prepare for it.

Your care of a specific patient or client: overviews

Review your current and recent work with this patient or client, consider any themes or threads which emerge and look at how you might apply your learning to working with this patient or client in the near future. Or consider your past work with this patient or client or similar patients/clients and consider what you have learned from your successes and mistakes. Anticipate your likely work with this patient or client or similar patients/clients right into the future and consider what you may need to do to develop yourself in your work with them.

Areas of responsibility in your work/caseload: specific incidents

Think back over the past few weeks at work and pick out some complicated situations you have been involved in, whether they went well or not so well. Identify any event that had an impact on you, whether you were concerned, upset or pleased about it. Or think further back in your time in this job or earlier in your career and notice any events that pop into your mind, even though they are long past. Notice especially those which have an emotional charge to them, for instance those in which you felt helpless, embarrassed, sad, angry, pleased with yourself, especially happy about your work, etc. You could scan back using any of these emotions as a theme, for instance: 'Times in my work when I've felt angry'.

Alternatively, think forward to any complex situations you will have to deal with soon and which you will have some responsibility for dealing with. Anticipate any major event which is likely to happen in years to come, which will affect your caseload or area of responsibility, such as planned organisational changes, a colleague leaving, etc.

Areas of responsibility in your work/caseload: overviews

Review your current and recent caseload/responsibilities and look at how you might set about managing them in the near future. Or consider your past caseload/responsibilities and how you managed them: reflect on what you have learned from your success and mistakes. Anticipate your likely caseload/responsibilities right into the future and consider what you may need to do to prepare yourself for managing them well.

Work and personal stresses and pressures: specific incidents

Pinpoint some recent occurrences at work which have resulted in your feeling stressed, or those outside work which may have influenced your concentration at work. Consider how you dealt with them and how you will handle them if they recur or their effects continue into the near future. Or scan further back in time and remember any stressful issues that affected your concentration or your feelings about your job, even though they are long past. Anticipate any additional work or personal stresses and pressures which are likely to occur in the future and consider how you might deal with them. These might include starting a new course, applying for promotion, moving on to another job in nursing, personal life events such as buying a house, children leaving home, retiring.

Work and personal stresses and pressures: overviews

Review the types of recent and current pressures of the job or personal stresses that may be influencing your concentration at work. Consider how you have been dealing with them in the past few weeks and how you will handle them in the next few weeks. Or think back over the types of work and personal stresses and pressures which have affected you in the past but which are now over. Alternatively, imagine the possible types of work or personal stresses and pressures which are likely to occur in the future and consider how you might deal with them.

Your development within your work: overviews

Consider what your job means to you at this stage in your life, what is important to you about doing this job rather than any other. Think about your recent development in your work, your feelings about it and where you seem to be going with it in the near future. Review your working career to date: pick out any themes or threads that seem to run through that time. Or, looking to your future, picture yourself in one, three or five or more years' time. Think about how ideally you would like your working life to be at that time, how you would like to feel about it, what kind of work you might be doing, what you need to do to make this come about.

Your development within your work: specific incidents

Focus on any recent incidents or people who have especially discouraged or inspired you in your development. Think back to earlier times in your career and recall incidents or people who especially discouraged or inspired you or consider turning points which resulted in your taking your present path. Imagine some likely changes and events in the future and consider how you might use them as learning opportunities for your own personal and professional development.

> David has worked on an elderly care ward for quite a few years and there are seldom any events which surprise him. When the time for his clinical supervision session approaches he often wonders what on earth he is going to talk about. Using this framework for the first time, he scans the diagram and the list of pointers and this gives him the idea to focus on his development within his work to date.

He begins to think back over the time he has been on the ward, what made him apply for the post, the changes he has experienced in the way the ward is run and what makes him stay in this post. He now has his first item for his clinical supervision session. Then he chooses to look at his relationship with one particular patient who has been on the ward for over a year and who seems to respond especially to David rather than anyone else. He now has two topics which could lead him to some in-depth reflection in his clinical supervision session.

If considering these options does not help you clarify something significant to reflect upon during clinical supervision then you probably have a mental block about it. The contributing factors to such a block are likely to be your unacknowledged emotional feelings. Perhaps you have some resentment about doing clinical supervision or specifically about your clinical supervisor or clinical supervision group. You may have unacknowledged fears to do with being criticised, or about lack of confidentiality and organisational links. Your feelings may be of unacknowledged sadness leading to your perhaps not wanting to let go of the past, such as a previous clinical supervisor or a previous job or nursing-as-it-used-to-be. It might be useful to bring to your clinical supervision your difficulty in thinking of issues and to discuss some of your feelings with your clinical supervisor or clinical supervision group. This might enable you to work through the block and become more able to prepare for and use the time available in clinical supervision. Clinical supervision is an ideal time and place to talk about your emotions and this is considered a sign of emotional competence, not a failing.

Begin reflecting before the session

Having identified some issues to bring to clinical supervision, you could begin to reflect on them using some of the intuitive and logical methods for reflection suggested in this chapter. During the session, your clinical supervisor may then be able to help you to deepen your reflection even further or to move on your thinking if you become stuck.

Intuitive methods of reflection

We offer some structures that may be helpful for making the transition between activity and reflection and you can use these before, during and after your clinical supervision sessions. They can be applied to any personal notes or reflective diary you might want to keep, to face-to-face work with your clinical supervisor or clinical supervision group or to any reflection you do as part of your professional practice.

Many of the methods for reflection identified in the nursing literature are based on frameworks for logical thinking, and have been developed by their authors to a level of complicated cognitive mapping which many nurses find daunting. We find that workshop participants are relieved and feel validated when we suggest that intuitive thinking skills are equally important.

Some issues require mainly one or other of the types of thinking skills; most demand a combination. Intuitive thinking can be useful when the issue you have to reflect upon is not clearcut: you may have incomplete information and cannot realistically get any more. In this type of situation, you are not clear what your goals are and it is not certain whether or not you will be able to achieve anything. The options open to you are not precise and you cannot easily predict the outcomes of any course of action. You can see from this that intuitive thinking can be especially useful when reflecting on complex and unpredictable issues involving emotions and human relationships.

Logical thinking on its own can be useful when the issue upon which you wish to reflect is fairly straightforward: when you have enough information about the problem, you can clarify what you are aiming at and it seems likely that you can at least in part achieve that aim. In this type of situation, the options open to you can be identified and you can more easily predict the outcomes of each option.

We find that the most frequent issues of concern that are brought to clinical supervision involve relationships with the patient/client, relatives, colleagues or managers. Applying a purely logical framework to trying to think these through would be a non-satisfying and ineffective process. Therefore we first suggest some intuitive methods of reflection which can be used on their own or combined with the more logical, sequential methods which follow. These intuitive methods are summarised in Table 4.1.

Table 4.1 Intuitive methods of reflection

- TOP-OF-THE-HEAD REFLECTION – Start talking or writing, without censoring; look back and pick out themes, significant points, gaps, steps in reflection so far
- FREE FALL WRITING – Write a 'stem' phrase at the top of a blank sheet; write anything, that comes into your mind, without censoring; stop at the end of time limit and look back; highlight one especially loaded phrase and write that at the top of another sheet as a new 'stem' phrase; continue; look back over your sheets and pick out any themes
- BRAINSTORMING – Write a specific question; within a time limit, list any ideas without censoring; rest; continue brainstorming for a further, shorter time limit; look back over all the ideas and cross out those which are totally out of the question; consider the others
- SLEEPING ON IT – Go to sleep at night thinking 'I wonder such and such . . .'; note any insights when you wake
- SHORT RELAXATION BREAK – Use physical relaxation techniques, 'time out' break to walk around or daydream or silence during the clinical supervision session, in order to allow intuitive thoughts to pop up
- DRAWING THE ISSUE – Ponder silently about the issue that you have identified; begin to draw freely in an abstract way, covering the paper; sit back and reflect on what you have drawn
- MIND MAPPING – Write a main heading; write the thoughts this heading stimulates, in a circle around the central point, linking each to the central heading with a line; expand on each of the thoughts by adding key words related to each one, in a little cluster around it; sit back and look at the overall map, noticing links

---

The most commonly used intuitive method is 'top-of-the-head reflection'. This is when you just start talking or writing about the issue and say whatever comes into your head about it, without censoring and without any deliberate order or structure. Then when you have run out of steam, look back over what you have said and try to pick out any themes, significant points that came out and surprised you or any gaps in your account that, in retrospect, you can see that you omitted. You might notice that you covered some of the steps in one or other of the logical reflection cycles. Your clinical supervisor or clinical supervision group can be helpful in helping you to identify the themes and logical steps you have already covered and the gaps in your thinking so far. Sometimes, the clinical supervisor may feel obliged to try to get you to organise your thoughts before you are ready, so it can be useful to warn her/him that you just want space to talk about it in your own words first before you marshal your thoughts.

A similar method is to write down an account of an issue using 'free fall writing' (Goldberg 1986). The technique is to set two time spans of, say, 2×7 minutes and write a 'stem' phrase at the top of a blank sheet, such as 'It all started when . . .' or 'I remember . . .'. Then for the first seven minutes, write absolutely anything that comes into your mind, without censoring, however much you think it sounds like rubbish. Keep writing for the whole of the time, do not lift your pen from the paper, do not think, do not correct or cross out. Then stop at the end of the time limit and look back over what you have written. Highlight one especially loaded phrase and write that at the top of another sheet as a new 'stem' phrase. Then do the second phase using the new 'stem' as a starting point for your seven minutes of 'free fall' writing. Then look back over your sheets and pick out any themes. This powerful method can feel like bungee-jumping on paper: a leap into thin air, not knowing where your thoughts will end up. It is therefore important to keep the contents of your sheets private, but to discuss the themes that emerged with your clinical supervisor or clinical supervision group if appropriate.

Brainstorming is probably the best known intuitive method. Write a specific question at the top of a sheet of paper, such as 'What are the factors which contribute to the problem?' or 'What are the options for dealing with the problem?' Set a time limit, say, five minutes. Within that time limit, make a list as quickly as you can of any idea at all that comes into your head: do not censor, but instead include any extreme, rude, dangerous, silly or ridiculous ideas that occur to you. After the time limit, take a few deep breaths and briefly scan the ideas, then continue brainstorming for a further, shorter time limit, say, two minutes. Look back over all the ideas and cross out those which are totally out of the question. Then consider the others. The aim of brainstorming is to loosen up your thinking, away from your usual train of thought towards more creativity. Although many of your ideas will need to be crossed out, these may have served the purpose of stimulating some useful ideas that you otherwise may not have considered. You can do this on your own or with your clinical supervisor: either of you could do the writing as you alone or both of you call out the brainstormed points. It is a useful method to use in clinical supervision groups to collect ideas and stimulate some mental energy.

Planning your agenda for your clinical supervision session at least 24 hours beforehand gives you the chance to sleep on it. 'Sleeping on it' is an intuitive skill which you can enhance by asking yourself a question, just before you go to sleep, beginning with 'I wonder . . .', such as 'I wonder what I'll say about that problem during clinical supervision tomorrow'. Then let your mind wander away from the topic, forget about it and go to sleep. When you wake or when you get to that issue in clinical supervision, sometimes some surprising insights can come to you without trying.

Sometimes letting yourself just relax allows intuitive thoughts to pop up. You can do this before the clinical supervision session, whether using relaxation techniques per se, or just having a 'time out' break to walk around or daydream. Don't strain to think about the problem, just let your mind drift. Sometimes an insight or a solution just begins to emerge if you let it. You can use silence during the clinical supervision session to allow ideas to emerge in this way.

Drawing the issue utilises and develops your capacity to think in pictures. Again, you can do this before the clinical supervision sessions and take your drawing along to discuss with your clinical supervisor or clinical supervision group, or you can take some pens and paper and do the drawing there. There are three steps: first of all ponder silently about the issue that you have identified. Begin to draw whilst you ponder and let your hand flow freely in an abstract way. Let the drawing develop until it covers the sheet of paper. Do not think about the drawing, or about whether or not you are producing a work of art. Just draw shapes and use colours whilst you think about the issue. You might want to include symbols or key words that mean something to you. Then you sit back and look at what you have drawn. Ask yourself what any of the parts of the drawing might symbolise about the issue or about yourself. Discuss this with your clinical supervisor or clinical supervision group. Anyone can use this method: even if you think you cannot draw, you will be able to doodle something about the issue in hand.

Using a mind map, first described by Buzan (1974) and developed by Buzan and Buzan (1995), is another effective intuitive method. It is based on the idea that thoughts arise out of the network of interconnections between the brain cells, not sequentially as if in a list. The electrical activity of the brain occurs so quickly that we cannot be conscious of every thought. You can slow down and capture some of these thoughts by recording them in a sort of map which takes into account how thoughts occur in the brain. Using a mind map to lay out your thoughts about an issue helps you to capture the range of thoughts you have about that issue, then to step back and look for themes and further connections.

Making a mind map has four stages. The first is to write a word or phase by way of a main heading, summarising the issue you want to think through, in the centre of a sheet of paper. Then write the thoughts this heading stimulates, in a circle around the central point, linking each to the central heading with a line. Third, expand on each of the thoughts by adding key words related to each one, in a little cluster around it. Then sit back and look at the overall map. Notice if any of the thoughts under separate sections link together, and draw a line across the page to link them. Add any further

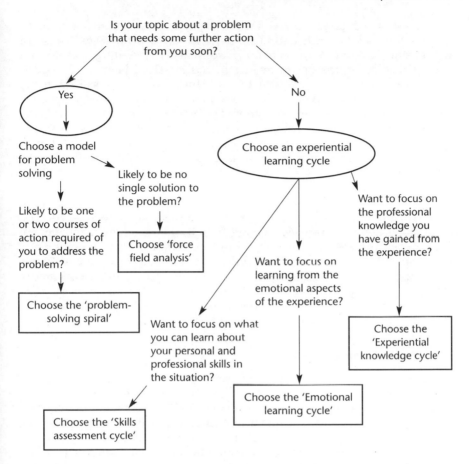

Figure 4.3 Choosing a logical model for reflection

thoughts that arise from each link. Emphasise any solutions or learning points, either in a different colour or with a bolder border. You can use this method as part of your preparation for clinical supervision and take the map to discuss with your clinical supervisor or clinical supervision group, or you can map it out during the clinical supervision session.

Intuitive methods on their own can be very successful or spectacularly unreliable: some crucial elements can be omitted. Using logical structures for reflection can help you to check that your intuitive thinking has taken everything into account. (See Figure 4.3.)

Logical frameworks for reflection

Part of the alienation which many nurses feel when trying to get to grips with published models for reflection may be due to what Davies (1995: 51) describes as 'masculine logic', which she suggests 'fears, denies and contains the world of bodily needs and emotions and interdependencies'. Much of the nursing literature on reflective practice makes dry reading, focusing on mainly analytic approaches to reflection, and the sheer plethora of models drives many nurses to 'analysis-paralysis': they cannot get started at all. Others try to cope by fixing on just one framework and trying to apply it, with inevitable difficulty, to every topic they wish to explore. To avoid being overwhelmed by the choice and complexity of models of reflection we recommend that as supervisee you first become aquainted with two different frameworks, one problem-solving framework and one experiential learning cycle, and use a simplified version of each to begin with. Then you can apply or combine them according to the issue in hand. As a rule of thumb, we suggest that you use a problem-solving framework when further action is going to be required from you in the future. When the issue is past and gone and you are wishing to reflect on your learning from it, then choose an experiential cycle. When you are adept at using both, you will be able to combine them for maximum effectiveness. Then you can expand your repertoire of frameworks for reflection by using a second problem-solving framework and a second experiential learning cycle and so on. As you become more familiar with your options, you could use the map in Figure 4.3 to help you choose a framework for each issue you want to explore.

Problem-solving frameworks

There are many structures for problem solving available to you, especially in books on management skills. We have adapted two which are of most interest to nurses attending our courses. The problem-solving spiral is useful when there are likely to be one or just a few courses of action required and the force field analysis is useful when there seems to be either nothing you can do about the problem or the contributing factors are so complex that you find it difficult to know where to start.

A problem-solving spiral

Figure 4.4 shows a step-by-step process of working through a problem to enable you to come to a clear decision. Although it is expressed in a certain sequence, you may have to take it in a slightly different order, or go back and forward until you are ready for the next step. For instance, having defined the problem and looked at contributing factors, you might realise that one of the contributing factors is the main problem that needs to be tackled first. In that case, you redefine that as the problem and then analyse the factors that contribute to it and move on through the cycle.

You can use some of the intuitive methods of reflection as part of this cycle. For instance, drawing the issue or mind mapping may be a good way of starting to define the problem and its contributing factors. Brainstorming is useful for considering options for action. This framework may highlight the steps you go through automatically when using intuitive methods such as 'top-of-the-head' reflection. However, we find that the most common pitfall for nurses is to go to the 'deciding on one option' stage too quickly, being anxious to

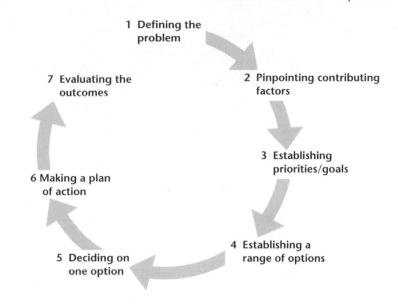

Figure 4.4 A problem-solving spiral

answer the question 'What am I going to do about it?' without thinking in depth first (see Figure 4.5). This framework can remind you not to skip important stages in reflection on a problem that you are keen to solve.

The following questions may help you to work your way through the spiral. A selection of questions is offered for each stage and it is important that you pick the one which seems most helpful to you: you do not have to answer every question. You can use these to enable you to pinpoint how far you have already thought through the problem, and how to deepen and move your thinking on. (See Figure 4.4.)

1 *Defining the problem*
   ● what's bothering you?
   ● what exactly is the problem for you?
   ● how do you feel about it?
2 *Pinpointing contributing factors*
   ● what do you think contributes to this problem or difficulty?
   ● how do you think you contribute to the problem?
   ● what's behind the problem?
   ● think of a time when this problem did not exist. What was different about the situation then?
   ● which of these factors do you think should be tackled first?
   ● do you need to redefine the problem or are you clear about what exactly the problem is?
3 *Establishing priorities/goals*
   ● what are you hoping to achieve?
   ● what are you hoping for/aiming at in the long run?

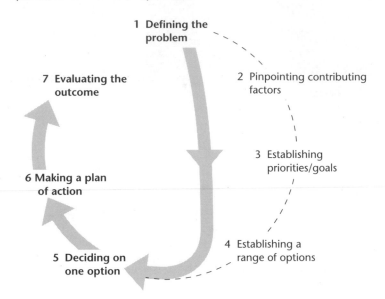

Figure 4.5 A common pitfall in problem solving

- imagine that it is now, say, six months later and this problem has been dealt with. What's different now?
- what are your ultimate goals?
- what short-term goals would help towards that end?
- are your goals realistic? If not, what would be more realistic?

4 *Establishing a range of options*
- what solutions have you tried already?
- what options have you thought of so far?
- allowing your ideas to flow freely, what ways can you think of to achieve your goals? Brainstorm and don't censor, just let anything, however crazy, come into your mind
- what's the most outrageous or extreme course of action that comes to mind? What's the most extreme form of inaction? Putting these two extremes at each end of a continuum, what options are there in between? Cross out anything which you are definitely not prepared to do under any circumstances whatsoever

5 *Deciding on one option*
- which is likely to be the most effective course of action, bearing in mind your goals?
- given that all your options are going to be difficult, which is the least worst?

6 *Making a plan of action*
- what's your plan?
- what is your very first step?
- then what next?
- whose help do you need?

- when exactly are you going to do these things?
- how will you keep up your courage and resolve to carry out this plan?
- how will you know if you have been successful?
- when exactly will you evaluate the outcome?

7 *(Later) Evaluating your decision*
- how far were your goals achieved?
- in the light of further information or events, what, if anything, needs to be done next?
- looking back at the factors contributing to the initial problem, is there anything else which could usefully be tackled?

Force field analysis

Force field analysis, first described by Lewin (1951), is a framework for dealing with a many-faceted problem for which there is no single solution. It is a useful structure for reflecting on many of the complex issues that you can bring to clinical supervision, especially when you feel stuck in trying to solve the problem. Figure 4.6 suggests a format to fill in for each step.

The first step is to describe the present situation – the 'frozen' or stuck position. Again, you might wish to use some intuitive methods such as mind mapping or drawing the issue to enable you to describe the complexity of the present situation. Then, for step 2, you need to take a leap of imagination and try to describe how you'd really like the situation to be – the 'vision'. (If you are writing or drawing this, use a different sheet of paper.) Try to include in your description the emotional tone and the relationship aspects of your vision, as well as any factual circumstances. Next, step 3 is to make a list of all the present factors which get in the way of your moving towards the vision: the restraining forces. Then, for step 4, ask yourself 'What are the present factors which would push the situation towards the vision if there were no restraining forces?' Alternatively, if it is hard to think so positively, ask yourself 'What factors prevent this situation being even worse?' – these are the driving forces.

Next consider how you can reduce the power of some of the restraining forces (step 5). Again, brainstorming can be an effective method of coming up with some creative ways of tackling these restraining forces. Write next to each one one small thing you can do to reduce its power. Then, for step 6, think about how you might enhance the power of the driving forces and write one small plan next to each point. You now have a detailed plan of a number of actions which will somewhat improve the situation.

Experiential learning cycles

Kolb (1984) first described a process of learning from experience: the experiential learning cycle. This has been much adapted since: here we outline some adaptations which focus on different elements of the learning experience: self-assessment of skills, personal professional knowledge and emotional learning. All experiential learning cycles have three fundamental stages of reflection as their core, which can be summarised under the headings: What?, So What? and Now What? (see Figure 4.7).

Step 4 Driving forces	Step 1 Frozen position	Step 3 Restraining forces		Step 2 Vision
List here	Describe here	List here		Describe here
1		1		
2		2		
3		3		
4		4		
5		5		
6		6		
7		7		
8		8		
Step 6 Plan steps to enhance the power of each driving force		**Step 5** Plan steps to reduce the power of each restraining force		

Figure 4.6   Force field analysis chart

The starting point for maximum learning from experience is to be fully engaged in the experience: to be involved with your concentration, emotions and active participation. Taking an observer role results in a relatively shallow experience and, correspondingly, a relatively superficial level of experiential learning. While there is a place for observing another experienced nurse at work in order to pick up tips about procedures or how to handle difficult situations, the deepest learning comes from the occasions when you yourself are fully involved in a situation. You can maximise your learning from experience by taking regular time to step back and reflect on

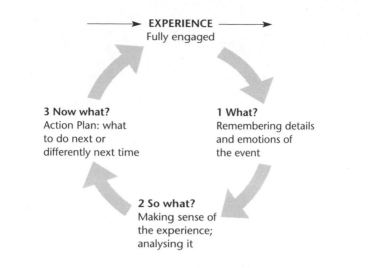

EXPERIENCE
Fully engaged

3 Now what?
Action Plan: what
to do next or
differently next time

1 What?
Remembering details
and emotions of
the event

2 So what?
Making sense of
the experience;
analysing it

Figure 4.7   Stages of a basic experiential learning cycle

significant experiences. Doing this with an experiential learning cycle to guide your thinking, and a clinical supervisor or clinical supervision group to help you deepen it, can enable you to continue building up your professional knowledge, expertise and realistic confidence as you deepen your knowledge of your patients/clients and yourself. Being able to monitor your practice by using an experiential learning cycle while you work, rather than only waiting for your clinical supervision sessions, is the ultimate aim in building these reflective skills.

Experiential learning cycles are frameworks to enable you to step back and look under the experience, analyse it and consider your learning from the experience and how you can apply that learning. During workshops, practice exercises and observations of real-life clinical supervision sessions, we see some common pitfalls which ensnare the supervisee into superficial reflection (see Figure 4.8). One is to stay preoccupied with recalling the event, going over and over the details without moving on to include the emotional dimension and analysing it in more detail to find its meaning and learning points. A second pitfall is to jump straight from the recall stage to the action planning stage, bypassing the in-depth reflection that is needed in order to discover the significance of the experience and your learning points. Both pitfalls are examples of avoidant, superficial reflection.

Some of the frameworks which follow may help you to deepen your reflection in each of the various stages of the experiential learning cycle. Each framework takes a slightly different focus.

A skills assessment cycle
This cycle may help you to make a self-assessment of the skills and abilities you used in the situation and how you can develop them in the future. It is especially useful for enabling you to practise taking a balanced view of the part you play in the complex situations you experience in your work. You

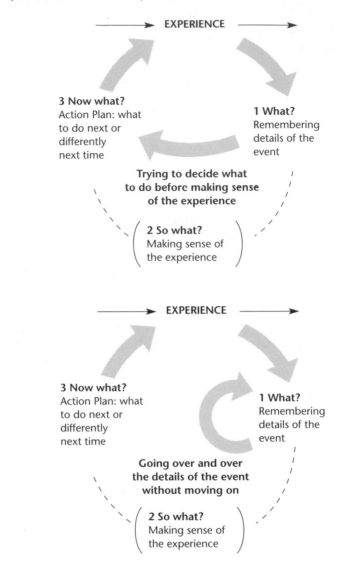

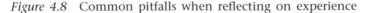

Figure 4.8   Common pitfalls when reflecting on experience

are encouraged to balance acknowledgement of your strengths with that of your weaknesses, and to consider how to use your strengths to greater effect as well as develop your areas of weakness. We find that nurses have a tendency to understate their strengths and overstate their weaknesses, although those who have been in a particular post for a long time can often go to the opposite extreme. Using this skills assessment cycle with your clinical supervisor or group can enable you to achieve and sustain a confidence about your expertise alongside an openness to learn. (See Figure 4.9.)

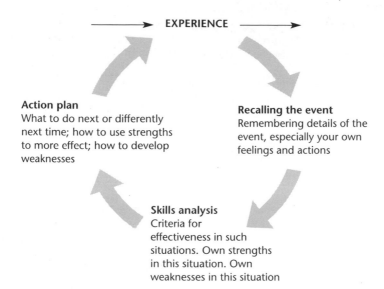

EXPERIENCE

Action plan
What to do next or differently next time; how to use strengths to more effect; how to develop weaknesses

Recalling the event
Remembering details of the event, especially your own feelings and actions

Skills analysis
Criteria for effectiveness in such situations. Own strengths in this situation. Own weaknesses in this situation

Figure 4.9 A skills assessment cycle

The following is a list of some pointers which might help you to reflect on the experience taking the focus of personal and professional skills. Again, the framework offers a selection of pointers for each stage: just pick the ones which seem most helpful in enabling you to deepen or move your thinking on.

Recalling the experience
- Describe the experience in your own words, in whatever sequence comes to you, putting the emphasis wherever you wish.
- If you haven't already, describe your own actions, thoughts and feelings at significant points.
- If you haven't already, pinpoint the reasons why you acted in the ways you did or why you failed to act.

Skills analysis
- Make a list of the professional and personal skills which would contribute to high quality practice in this type of situation. Put as many as you can into your list of criteria for excellence (minimum number: 15). Ensure that you write a phrase or sentence about each one, because single word criteria are usually too general.
- Include a wide range of professional skills, such as those which come within the categories of: technical, interpersonal, care planning, team work, health education, support, staff education and so on.
- Include a wide range of personal skills, such as those which come within the categories of: time management, stress management, self-assessment, reflection, problem solving, decision making, emotional skills and so on.

- Looking at this list, pick out one which was one of your strengths in this situation. If you cannot think of anything positive, if perhaps your confidence is having a bad day, pick one at which you think you were least hopeless!
- Then select one criterion from the list which was one of your weaknesses in this situation. If you cannot think of anything in terms of a weakness, perhaps because your humility is having a bad day, then select one at which you were least perfect!
- Repeat the last two steps until you have three of each type of criterion: three strengths and three weaknesses. Ensure that you have an equal number of strengths and weaknesses.

Action plan
- Make a step-by-step plan of how you are going to develop one of your strengths and one of your weaknesses.
- Make a similar plan for the other strengths and weaknesses.
- Outline how you hope to apply this development should you ever be in a similar situation again: what would you do differently?

A personal/professional knowledge cycle of experiential learning
Johns (1994) has utilised some of Carper's (1978) work on four ways of knowing, and incorporated it into this experiential learning cycle. Johns' cycle is especially useful for building your awareness of and confidence in the professional knowledge that you develop from personal involvement in the experience of working with a patient. He suggests that the emphasis on research-based practice has become too extreme. This has devalued the knowledge nurses gain from their own experience and those areas of nursing practice which cannot be easily measured, such as compassion, caring, motivation, intuition, personal and interpersonal skills and so on. Johns takes a 'new paradigm' stance on research: that using any of the experiential learning cycles in order to enquire into one's own personal professional knowledge is a valid method of research – see Reason and Rowan (1981) for an account of this.

Figure 4.10 shows our adaptation of Johns' cycle. We follow his cue questions to lead you through the process. Again, the list gives a selection of questions for each stage: you would not be expected to try to answer them all. Use them to identify how far you have got already in your thinking, then pick out only the ones which help you to think more deeply or move on.

Questions to guide you through the personal professional knowledge cycle are taken from Johns (1994: 112):

Core question: *'What information do I need access to in order to learn through this experience?'*
1 *Description of the experience*
- Phenomenon – describe the 'here and now' experience
- Causal – what essential factors contributed to this experience?
- Context – what are the significant background factors to this experience?
- Clarifying – what are the key processes (for reflection) in this experience?

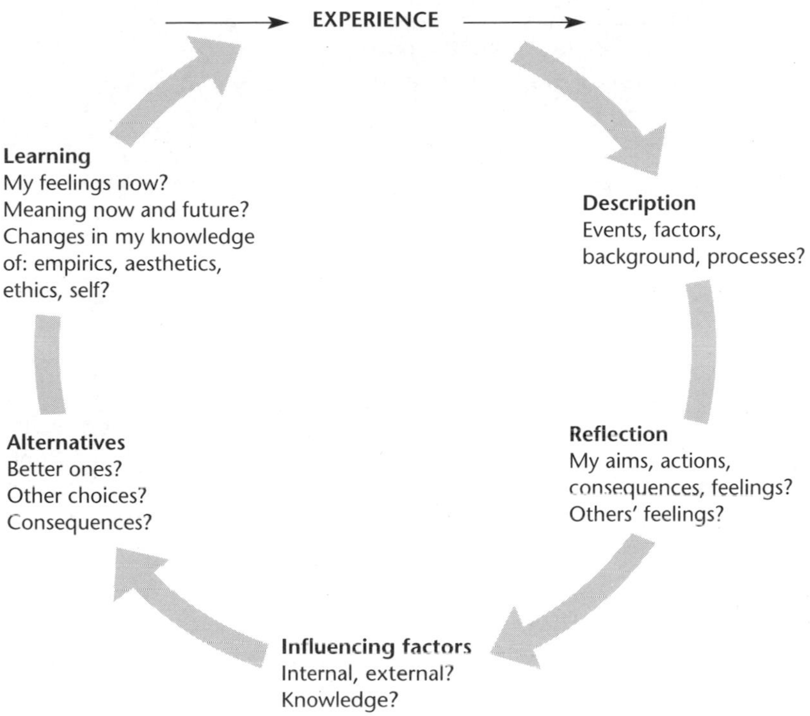

EXPERIENCE

Learning
My feelings now?
Meaning now and future?
Changes in my knowledge
of: empirics, aesthetics,
ethics, self?

Description
Events, factors,
background, processes?

Alternatives
Better ones?
Other choices?
Consequences?

Reflection
My aims, actions,
consequences, feelings?
Others' feelings?

Influencing factors
Internal, external?
Knowledge?

Figure 4.10 A personal/professional knowledge cycle (after Johns 1994)

2 *Reflection*
- What was I trying to achieve?
- Why did I intervene as I did?
- What were the consequences of my actions for:
  - myself?
  - the patient/family?
  - the people I work with?
- How did I feel about this experience when it was happening?
- How did the patient feel about it?
- How do I know how the patient felt about it?

3 *Influencing factors*
- What internal factors influenced my decision making?
- What external factors influenced my decision making?
- What sources of knowledge did influence/should have influenced my decision making?

4 *Could I have dealt better with the situation?*
- What other choices did I have?
- What would have been the consequences of these choices?

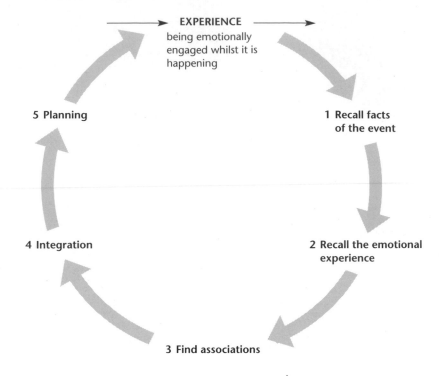

Figure 4.11   Emotional skills cycle

5 *Learning*
  ● How do I feel now about this experience?
  ● How can I make sense of this experience in the light of past experi-
    ences and future practice?
  ● How has this experience changed my ways of knowing: empirics
    (the science of nursing); aesthetics (the art of nursing); ethics (the
    moral component of nursing); personal (self-knowledge)?

An emotional skills learning cycle
We aim to demystify the emotional element of clinical supervision and
ensure that it has its place alongside professional knowledge and skills as
worthy of examination. This emotional skills development framework may
help you to reflect on what can be learned about your abilities in using your
emotional energy (see Figure 4.11). It includes some adapted elements from
Boud *et al.*'s (1985) framework of reflection in learning.

   We suggest some pointers which might help you to reflect on the experience with the focus on emotional skills. Again, use the framework to aug-
ment your existing thinking about the experience and to highlight any
stages you have left out in your reflection so far or that you need to explore
in more depth. Pick the pointers which seem most helpful to you.

Questions and prompts to guide you through the emotional skills cycle:

1 *Recall the facts of the event*
   - describe the sequence of events as factually as you can without interpreting or analysing them at this point and without describing your feelings

2 *Recall the emotional experience*
   - describe the whole experience, or the most important part of the experience, again, but this time in the present tense
   - what kind of atmosphere do you pick up?
   - what colours, tone, sounds, sensations do you notice in particular?
   - what are you thinking?
   - how are you feeling?
   - what do your feelings lead you to do?
   - how do your emotional feelings help or hinder you in this situation?
   - what emotional skills did you use?

3 *Find associations*
   Use any of the intuitive methods shown earlier in the chapter to discover associations: 'top of the head' reflection; free fall writing; drawing the issue; mind mapping, brainstorming. Do not censor. Whilst you are doing this, consider these questions and include your answers in the account:
   - what does this situation remind you of?
   - when have you felt like this before?
   - taking each of the emotions you identified in Stage 2, brainstorm associations using the seed phrase 'Times I've felt . . .'

4 *Integration*
   - what themes or linking patterns can you see?
   - how did your emotion positively and negatively affect your actions?
   - what conclusions do you draw from reviewing the emotional content of the experience like this?

5 *Planning*
   - make a step-by-step plan that is possible and realistic
   - how will you apply these conclusions now?
   - how might you apply these conclusions in future?
   - with whose help?
   - what emotional skills will you use?
   - rehearse how you will apply them: either by talking through the sequence of action; writing it down; setting up a role play with your clinical supervisor or clinical supervision group or a colleague
   - when and how will you review your plan?

Concepts such as 'emotional competence' (Heron 1983) and 'emotional skills' (Bond 1986) have been used for some time and are gaining ground, along with 'positive emotional processes' (Heron 1989), 'emotional literacy' and 'emotional intelligence' (Goleman 1996). The emotional learning cycle will be particularly useful to you if you are familiar with frameworks for understanding emotions and practical methods of building emotional skills.

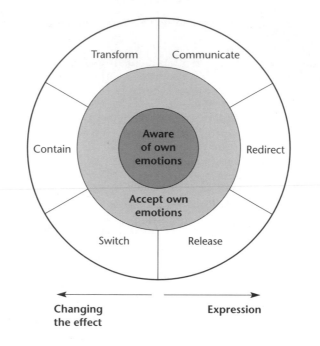

Figure 4.12   Emotional skills

Emotional skills can be learned and developed. There is a common mis-conception that once a person reaches a state of 'maturity', they have learned all they can about emotions. However, just as you can develop new technical or intellectual skills, you can go on building your emotional skills. These emotional skills can be summarised as shown in the diagram in Figure 4.12, a framework adapted from Heron's (1989) 'positive emotional processes'. Emotional skills can be described as the two central skills of awareness and self-acceptance, from which emerge the skills of being able to change the effect of emotional impulses (containment, switching, transformation) and the skills of emotional expression (communication, redirection and release).

Awareness involves noticing your own emotions, being able to identify them and note the extent to which they can positively and negatively influence your behaviour. This is essential for being able to selectively control emotional impulses rather than put a blanket repression on all of them. This leaves room for choice about expressing emotions and using them as a resource as well as containing them. One way of becoming more aware of your emotions is to notice their physical effects: a sensation of energy, tingling, alertness can tell you that you are interested, motivated, excited, pleased or delighted. Warmness in the chest and arms may indicate liking and affection whilst heaviness in the chest may be sadness, grief or despair. Tensions in the jaw and shoulders may indicate irritation, resentment or anger. Stomach churning, lower back tensions, unpleasant tingling, tightness in the chest or fidgety legs may tell you that you are worried, anxious or fearful.

Non-critical acceptance of the existence of your emotions is important though difficult in the culture of the health service. It involves not blaming or crediting the feelings on someone else, and not being critical with yourself for having them. Awareness and acceptance go hand in hand. The more you can come to accept your feelings non-judgementally, the easier it will become to be increasingly aware of your emotions and the energy that goes with them. Repression and suppression take up a lot of energy and can leave you feeling exhausted, whereas awareness and acceptance of emotions liberates energy which you can use positively. Using clinical supervision to put your feelings into words can help develop your self-acceptance provided your clinical supervisor can listen non-judgementally.

Redirection is the skill of channelling the energy of emotions into constructive thought or action. For instance, if your ability to do your work is hindered by a certain Trust policy and you are in danger of blowing your top if you try to challenge the system, you could temporarily divert the energy of the frustration away from the problem and channel it into getting a lot of office or household chores done quickly. Then when you have calmed down a little, you could use the energy to tackle the problem constructively, perhaps by getting together with colleagues to collect evidence and go through the correct channels to suggest a change of policy.

Communication about your emotions helps to reduce superficiality and build trust in relationships. It includes taking the risk of sharing positive feelings, revealing emotional vulnerability and giving constructive criticism. Verbal communication about emotions requires you to be emotionally articulate, to have a vocabulary of words that you can draw on to describe the feelings you experience. Communication may also be in a creative form such as poetry, dance, painting, drawing, music, etc.

Emotional release is a controlled process of letting go. You are aware of what you are doing and choosing to do it safely at the appropriate time and place. It may involve yelling, bashing cushions, crying, sobbing, trembling, laughing or putting a lot of strength of feeling into verbal communication about emotions. You need to choose times of privacy or times with non-judgemental family, friends or colleagues with whom you can release feelings from time to time. Clinical supervision may be an appropriate place for short periods of letting off steam. We have found nurses often feel ashamed at crying in clinical supervision sessions but are relieved when it is pointed out that they are actually using an emotional skill by choosing an appropriate time and place to do this.

Containment is about holding back or holding onto emotions. There are many occasions when you need to hold back, perhaps to avoid hurting someone or when people are depending on you to act efficiently. The usually accepted concept of control is a sort of grit-your-teeth-holding-back-the-reins, which is ultimately exhausting. Containment is about expanding your sense of your own personal strength so that you can contain the feelings, gently 'holding' that part of you which is feeling emotional and postponing expressing the feelings until a more appropriate time. Earlier in this book we referred to the containing function of clinical supervision where we can name and acknowledge anxieties and the inner conflicts they can produce.

Nurses who have good clinical supervision speak of the containing effect of just knowing they can rely on getting their time and how much this helps them to contain some of the difficult feelings triggered by day-to-day work.

Switching is when you get yourself into a different emotional state by positive self-talk, doing something neutral like making a cup of tea or taking a 'time out' break to get a change of environment to change your mood.

Transformation is a difficult process to describe and, for some, difficult to experience as it usually relates to a more spiritual side of a person, which not everyone would choose to address. It is a meditative process of going into the emotions and feeling them intensely until your experience takes you through them to an altered state of consciousness. Most religions have prayers or meditations which can enable transformation of emotions and there are secular techniques of relaxation and meditation which serve this purpose.

For further guidance about practical ways of building emotional skills, you may wish to refer to guidelines we have provided elsewhere, such as in Bond (1986, 1989) and Holland (1987). Some stress management books address this issue, though not all view emotions as such potentially positive resources.

In Chapter 2 we suggested that although clinical supervision provides an important space for feelings to surface, uncomfortable or painful emotions cannot always be magically removed or made better, however much we may unconsciously want to rescue and repair. For example, feelings of grief and loss need to be replayed and relived over and over before the intensity can lessen. Developing your emotional skills enables you to use clinical supervision and any other appropriate setting for giving air time to both celebratory and uncomfortable feelings and releasing the positive energy that they generate.

Developmental stages in using clinical supervision skills

As with any other set of skills, as supervisee, you will learn from the experience of using the time offered in clinical supervision. As your skills, confidence in yourself and trust in your clinical supervisor develop, you will be able increasingly to deepen your reflective process during clinical supervision sessions. The 'So What?' phase of the experiential learning cycle will become deeper and your ability to put into practice what you have learned from reflection will be increasingly effective. You will find yourself being more and more able to use the support and guidance of the clinical supervisor or clinical supervision group and to give yourself this type of support and guidance whilst you are working in practice.

Stages in reflection on client/patient care

You will notice your development in the way you reflect about your care of specific patients or clients. Figure 4.13 suggests some phases through which you may progress.

This framework is adapted from an idea by Hawkins and Shohet (1989) and is based on our observations of clinical supervision practice sessions

Level 1	Level 2	Level 3	Level 4
Focus: Problem-centred	(Includes Level 1) *Focus:* Client/patient centred	(Includes Level 1)	(Includes Level 1)
Key question: 'Am I doing the right thing?' 'What do I do next?'		(Includes Level 2)	(Includes Level 2)
Level 1	*Key question:* 'How is the client/patient developing?'	*Focus:* Relationship with client/patient	(Includes Level 3) *Focus:* Developing the 'internal supervisor'
	Level 2	*Key question:* 'How am I and the client/patient relating and what's my part in that?'	*Key question:* 'What am I learning about being reflective while I am actually working with the client/patient?'
		Level 3	
			Level 4

Figure 4.13 Developmental stages in using clinical supervision as supervisee

during courses and some real-life clinical supervision sessions, but is suggested tentatively. Although we have tended to see these stages according to the length of time the supervisee has been receiving clinical supervision, some individuals may start at a different point. For some, the focus of Level 4 may be the easier starting point, yet they may not have highly developed problem-solving skills. A danger that we see in using such a developmental framework is that some nurses can apply a hierarchy of value to the stages: diminishing the importance of, say, problem solving, when they have achieved the dizzy heights of Level 4: a competitive 'I'm-more-self-aware-therefore-a-better-person-than-my-problem-solving,-practically-oriented-colleagues' approach. We maintain that all stages in the framework are important and no early stage should be abandoned in favour of the later stages.

The internal supervisor

The term 'internal supervisor' was coined by Patrick Casement with reference to the needs of trainees in counselling and psychotherapy, but it is also relevant and applicable to the process of clinical supervision in nursing. This is a fairly advanced part of the reflective process and needs to be developed

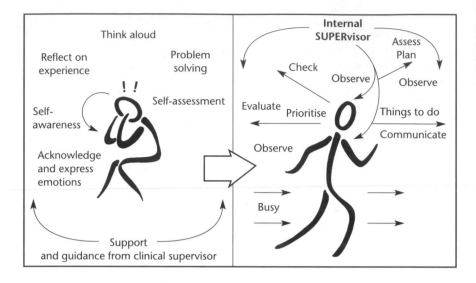

Figure 4.14 Transition from reflection ON practice to reflection IN practice

slowly over a period of time, moving from an initial focus on specific incidents or problems to a continuous internalised reflection and supervision by you as supervisee about your own skills, perceptions, understanding of and relationship with your client. This mirrors the concept of 'learning through practice' as described by Fish *et al.* (1989). Casement describes the developmental process well; we change the words slightly to adapt it to clinical supervision in nursing:

> At the outset, [supervisees] may rely a good deal upon the advice and comments offered by the supervisor. With time these supervisory insights should become more integrated in to the on-going work [with clients] . . . During the course of being supervised, [supervisees] need to acquire their own capacity for spontaneous reflection within the session . . . they can learn to watch themselves as well as the [client], now using this island of intellectual contemplation and mental space within which their internal supervisor [the skills acquired and absorbed in supervision] can begin to operate.
>
> (Casement 1985: 32)

The time you spend reflecting *on* practice during your clinical supervision sessions enables you to build and deepen your skills of reflecting *in* practice, as illustrated in Figure 4.14.

Implicit in these skills is your capacity as supervisee to be in two places at once, in the shoes of your client, and at the same time having your feet firmly embedded in your own footwear. This is what makes it different from more cognitive self-analysis as the ability to empathise, feel and respond using your intuitive skills is vital to this interactive process which includes rather than excludes the client. It can prevent what Davies (1995) continues to see as a problem in Schön's (1983) framework of reflective practice, namely the continued professional emotional distance from the client. Although 'internal supervision' is about the ability to stand apart, from both yourself and from your client, you are still engaged in the process of interacting with the client whilst monitoring the relationship between you. Swain (1995) reminds us that it is not the same as standing aloof or disengaging, as this would severely damage our clinical responsiveness. But you can use this heightened awareness of your own inner responses to develop and improve your attentiveness and effectiveness at the same time as being attentive to the patient.

We hope this chapter has been a helpful resource from which to select some frameworks to aid your reflection during clinical supervision sessions. Your taking the initiative in using these frameworks will give you the power you require to make full use of the clinical supervision relationship, to lead the sessions and ensure your time is spent on your own in-depth reflection on your practice and the part you play as an individual in the complexity and quality of your practice. We hope also that it has been useful to highlight the longer-term, ongoing development of your skills of reflection-in-practice as a result of your experiences as a supervisee. The next two chapters are addressed to clinical supervisors and members of clinical supervision groups, but even if you do not fall into either category, they may yet cover some useful ground to illustrate what you might expect from your clinical supervisor.

Support and catalytic skills
of the clinical supervisor

The clinical supervisor is expected to emphasise the 'power to' aspects of the power relationship, seeking to empower the supervisee and use enabling skills in which are embraced all the main principles of clinical supervision. The supportive and formative elements are the main means by which the normative function is carried out. This chapter will focus on these supportive and formative elements but these need to be balanced with normative too, seen within the context of the working alliance between supervisee and clinical supervisor and within the organisational setting. Chapter 6 addresses the more authoritative aspects of the clinical supervisor's role more specifically, but in looking here in more depth at the support and catalytic skills of the clinical supervisor, we need to bear in mind that the aim of clinical supervision is the development and maintenance of quality practice.

In this and the next chapter, we refer to the clinical supervisor mainly in the context of one-to-one clinical supervision. However, we wish to emphasise that these skills are also necessary for all members of a clinical supervision group; Chapter 7 places this in context.

A framework for exploring the enabling skills of the clinical supervisor

Dartington (1994: 101), in her study on idealism and despondency in hospital nursing, suggests that 'What is usually absent is the opportunity to ask the question "Why?" of someone in authority, someone who is not surprised by the questions, who is interested in the answer and who can engage in a spirit of mutual enquiry.' For this spirit of mutual enquiry it will need someone to ask and someone to respond. Through using support and catalytic skills, the clinical supervisor can be the person to provide the opportunity for this mutual enquiry into the many complex aspects of practice for which there are no straightforward answers.

The next two chapters focus on specific helping skills of the clinical supervisor. Much of what we have written will look familiar to you since these skills are already an intrinsic part of your work in any helping relationship, whether with patients, clients, colleagues, students, your own friends or family. We find that workshop participants gain from identifying these helping skills and applying them to clinical supervision. We seek to give you the chance to identify your own strengths and weaknesses.

We looked at the concepts and skills of reflection in Chapter 4 and in the next two chapters we focus on the facilitation skills of the clinical supervisor and clinical supervision group member. Before we identify the nature of these skills, it might be useful to clarify the meaning of 'facilitate'. Dictionary definitions are: 'To free from difficulties and obstacles, to make easy'; 'To lessen the labour of, assist (a person)', 'To render easier, to promote, help forward' (*Shorter Oxford Dictionary* 1983). There may be a contradiction in the use of the word 'facilitate' in this respect: sometimes it would 'lessen the labour of, assist, render easier, promote, help forward' to do the task *for* the person(s). That is, it can seem *more* difficult or laborious on the receiving end to have someone enable you to do something for yourself rather than tell you the answer or do it for you.

The word 'facilitate' has come to mean, in many areas of professional communication, to supportively enable another person or group of people to do or learn something for themselves, rather than doing it for them. Underpinning this is the belief that enabling the other to achieve their goal themselves not only gets the task done, but increases their sense of ownership of the outcome, and provides a learning experience which can contribute positively to self-development and increased effectiveness in the future. Or as the Chinese proverb says: 'Give a man a fish and you feed him for one day: teach him how to fish and you feed him for many days'. Jacques (1991: 124) describes facilitation: 'It involves careful listening and eliciting rather than giving one's own knowledge . . . It should not be supposed that the facilitator role represents a "laissez-faire" style of leadership: rather is there a sense of shared or developed responsibility for learning'.

In our framework, we identify four main types of facilitation skills: supportive, catalytic, informative and challenging. (See Figure 5.1.) These have similarities to Heron's (1990) six-category intervention analysis (prescriptive,

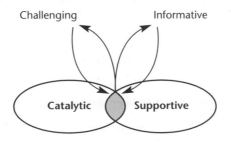

Figure 5.1 Four main skills of the clinical supervisor

informative, confronting, cathartic, catalytic and supportive) and the intervention styles described by Cockman *et al.* (1992) (acceptant, catalytic, confrontational and prescriptive).

Each of these four types of skills depends on your intention: that is, what you intend as far as your communication with the supervisee is concerned. This framework does not indicate that any one of these is 'better' than another. Any helping relationship will need to include a mixture of these four skills of communication; the relative balance between the four types of communication is defined by the type of relationship, its purpose and any agreed contract between the people involved.

As a clinical supervisor, your aim is to achieve an appropriate balance by using mainly the non-directive (supportive and catalytic) interventions: these are the heart of your communication in clinical supervision. The more directive (informative and challenging) interventions very occasionally arise from and quickly return to your non-directive communication base. This might be in contrast to, say, a preceptor who is working with a newly qualified nurse taking up her first post in a unit new to her, when the preceptor may need to define more of the agenda and pass on a body of information because she has more knowledge of what needs to be covered. As another contrasting example, a team manager who is meeting with a team member to apply a management-by-objectives approach would use more directive skills in outlining organisational and team objectives and challenging any lack of achieving them, in addition to drawing out the team member's own objectives within that framework. The clinical supervisor's approach should be more focused on the supervisee's agenda and on mostly non-directive facilitation of the exploration of those topics.

Many of the pitfalls in facilitating the supervisee arise from:

- a genuine desire to show that you are listening and that you are wanting to help, but the type of support turns out to be inappropriate
- lack of knowledge of ways of showing explicit support
- lack of skill
- lack of awareness of your own uncontained feelings of anxiety, helplessness, embarrassment or frustration
- lack of skill in containing or expressing your own feelings when you are aware of them.

This chapter highlights some aspects of support and catalytic facilitation that especially apply to the clinical supervision situation. These non-directive skills of the clinical supervisor are the bedrock of the relationship. There are some similarities between this aspect of clinical supervision and counselling, but also some crucial differences.

Distinguishing between clinical supervision and counselling

Many of the skills outlined in this section will be familiar to you, possibly reminiscent of counselling skills training sessions. It is important, however, to be clear about the difference between clinical supervision and counselling. Table 5.1 highlights some of the differences.

Following through your intention to take a non-directive or directive approach requires conscious and intuitive use of specific skills. Many clinical supervisors assess themselves as being strongest at supporting and giving information, and less strong at challenging. So, perhaps starting with one of your strengths, we'll start looking at the supportive skills of clinical supervision.

The rest of this chapter aims to help you to:

- give names to the skills of support and catalytic facilitation that you already use
- relate them to your role as clinical supervisor
- clarify your supportive and catalytic intentions and your options for putting those intentions into practice
- pinpoint some of the pitfalls that you might fall into when intending to be supportive and catalytic, and clarifying some ways of avoiding these pitfalls.

Support skills of the clinical supervisor

As Swain (1995: 29) points out, there is still a need for staff support, peer support, and 'courteous, sensitive, consultative organisational management': clinical supervision should not replace any of these. She goes on to say: 'That said, a support element is intrinsic to the clinical supervision process. This, while not "cosy", should be holding; while not counselling in a formal sense, will be listening to the individual's "feeling state", as she carries out her work, and will use counselling skills; while not occupational health, will take note of the supervisee's "health" state.'

Be explicitly supportive

Your relationship as a clinical supervisor needs to be fundamentally supportive at all times. The time available in clinical supervision is short and it is important to find ways of showing support openly and explicitly so that the supervisee can quickly recognise the support that is available. However, one common pitfall in setting out intentionally to be supportive is to lack genuineness. To find what exactly you can be genuine about, it can be helpful to identify exactly what it is that you are supporting about the person.

When working with a supervisee whom you find difficult genuinely to support, referring to the points shown in Figure 5.2 might help. Consider something about them that you can focus on, to build the supportive element in the relationship. Any catalytic work, information or advice giving or challenging you do needs to be based on some genuine support for that person.

For instance, you may be appalled at the way a supervisee describes going about handling a situation, the way she speaks in a derogatory manner about other staff and diminishes their contributions and worth. However,

Table 5.1   Distinguishing between counselling and clinical supervision

	Counselling	Clinical supervision
Agenda	Agenda defined by the supervisee	Agenda mostly defined by the supervisee. Clinical supervisor may add items arising during the sessions or refocus on how any personal issues discussed affect practice
Confidentiality	Total, with legal exceptions. Counsellor may keep own records that are absolutely confidential	Almost total, with exceptions of legal or professional ethics. Record may be made to pass on within the organisation of attendance dates and times. Record of content may be negotiated between practitioner and clinical supervisor, for their eyes only
Information from facilitator	Information, advice or guidance very rarely given, and then usually focused on emotional issues	Some information, advice, guidance offered to supplement the supervisee's own expertise, to help the supervisee see options available and make own informed decision
Challenge from facilitator	Non-judgemental about the person's emotional issues. Very occasional challenges about defences against emotional expression and growth	Challenging technical mistakes, inadequate clinical standards, contribution to problems with team work, more personal issues such as unhelpful or self-defeating behaviour or attitude, blind spots, broken contracts. Based on evidence gained during the clinical supervision session
Support from facilitator	Support for the client as a person, often especially for emotional awareness and expression. Support is open-ended	Support for the supervisee as a person and encouragement given to help supervisee recognise and use own expertise and personal abilities towards developing their professional expertise. Any exploration of personal issues eventually related back to how these affect practice. Clinical supervisor acknowledges any emotional issues about the past which are disclosed, but suggests that her/his remit is to help with the present-day feelings and practicalities
Catalytic help from facilitator	Enabling reflection and problem solving in the direction of deeper exploration into the personal and relationship aspects of the problem, including the transference relationship between client and counsellor	Enabling reflection on issues ultimately affecting practice (including some consideration of issues involved in the clinical supervision relationship), learning from experience, problem solving, pinpointing ways of dealing with difficult emotions, decision making and planning. All of these with the ultimate emphasis on reviewing application to practice

Emotions and their level
of intensity

Needs as a professional

Needs a human being

Goals, priorities, vision,
hopes for the future

Their perception of the
situation

Experience of the
pressures they are under

Vulnerabilities

Intention

Specific behaviour, actions
approach or manner

Motivation, commitment

Rights in terms of the post
they hold and especially
rights as a human being

Specific values, principles

Particular qualities,
achievements

Figure 5.2 Be specific about what you are supporting about the supervisee

before you tackle your concerns, you explore the pressures she is under, the commitment she has to making it work, and show support for her in these respects. Only when you sense she really does feel supported by you, that you are on her side (though not colluding or agreeing with her mistakes), do you begin to enable her to look at more effective ways of handling the situation, and challenge her if she seems unwilling to change her approach.

Figure 5.2 suggests some specific aspects of the supervisee that you may be able to support: we have identified these examples to enable you to express explicit support in a very specific way. Sometimes you genuinely feel that you can support one aspect, but not another: for instance, you can support the supervisee's good intentions to help a client but you cannot support the way she is going about it. We are not suggesting that when you are concerned about something you seek something positive to say first, then add the challenge with a 'but'. We are advocating letting explicit support stand on its own. When we come to the section on challenging, we will also advocate that a challenge stands on its own without sugaring the pill.

Ways of showing support

In the next part of this chapter, we will give illustrations of ways of showing support that might apply to the following example, so, to set the scene, it is introduced here.

Sharma is telling her clinical supervisor, Pat, about a traumatic incident in her ward, of which she is the manager. The relative of a very ill patient had been physically violent with another relative, causing a severe injury, and verbally violent and threatening towards staff. The details of the incident are shocking and Sharma recounts everything she did to deal with the situation at the time: follow-up

Table 5.2 Ways of showing support in clinical supervision

- RELIABILITY AND PUNCTUALITY – Making appointments with supervisee a priority; being punctual and sticking to time boundaries
- SETTLING – Enabling the supervisee to settle, relax and put their journey to the session behind them (you need to be composed, settled and relaxed yourself first!)
- SHOWING YOU ARE LISTENING WITH ACCEPTANCE – Paying attention to the supervisee as a human being and seeking to understand the supervisee's perception of the situation they are describing; showing you are listening by your non-verbal responses and by summarising their viewpoint, respecting it as their perspective
- ENCOURAGEMENT – Showing interest, pointing out strengths or achievements that the supervisee has shown, encourage the supervisee to talk positively about herself
- TUNING IN – Tuning in to the emotions being expressed or which are implicit and tuning in to their level of intensity; putting into words and acknowledging the level of emotion that underlies what supervisee is saying; tentatively to allow supervisee to find their own words for their feelings; accepting of the emotion, non-critical
- ADVOCACY – Indicating that the supervisee deserves better, perhaps more consideration, information, respect for personal or professional rights, support, etc.
- SUPPORTIVE SILENCE – Space to reflect
- GIVING PERMISSION FOR EMOTIONAL RELEASE – Supporting emotional release without making a fuss; giving permission to show your acceptance
- ENABLING EMOTIONAL RECOVERY – When the supervisee is ready, distracting attention away from feelings and refocusing on reflection and problem solving
- SELF-DISCLOSURE – Sharing a little of your own experience or feelings; expressing any caring and concerned feelings you have about the supervisee
- APOLOGISING – For any of your mistakes, without defensiveness

liaison with the police and the support for her staff and future planning to prepare them better in future for such events. She is anxiously asking Pat to tell her where she went wrong, what else she could have done or should be doing now.

We will return to this example later.

We suggest eleven distinct ways of showing support explicitly through your actions, your manner and what you say (see Table 5.2). First, a clinical supervisor needs to be reliable. It is important to make appointments with your supervisee a priority, only postponing or cancelling them in dire emergencies. The planned, regular protected time gives a regular structure to the support the supervisee experiences from clinical supervision. This psychological holding is almost as important as the process of the session itself and meets some of the human need for security in the workplace which we discussed in Chapter 2. A practitioner who knows she can rely on the regular sessions is more able to contain the stresses and distresses of their work. Punctuality in starting and finishing the session is part of this structure of support. By repeatedly sticking to the agreed time boundaries you are building the supervisee's responsibility and ability to use the time effectively. If you find there are other pressures in your own work that might lead you to postpone, cancel or be late for sessions, then you need to consider whether being a clinical supervisor is appropriate to your role in the organisation. Many managers attending our workshops find that they are so often called to emergency management meetings or to deal with management crises that the clinical supervision they can offer is only a haphazard, low priority affair.

Your first supportive task in a clinical supervision session is to enable the supervisee to settle into the session, to make the often difficult adjustment from the busy-ness of action-oriented work to sitting and reflecting. Your relaxed, thoughtful manner at the beginning of a session can be very supportive in enabling this transition. In practical terms, this means you need to settle yourself, taking a few minutes of undisturbed time before the session to put aside your other preoccupations, and to focus your thoughts on the individual with whom you are about to work.

A clinical supervisor needs to be able to listen with acceptance, paying attention to the supervisee as a human being, giving space for them to find their own words. Showing that you are listening by your non-verbal responses is important, not only giving good eye contact, but reacting with your facial and body expression and with non-verbal sounds such as 'hm' to the supervisee's emphatic points. You listen not only to the words but also to tone, real meanings, emotions, the supervisee's own perception of the situation they are describing. Your listening needs to be active, proving that you are listening by your occasional attempts to summarise what the supervisee is saying. This summary can be experienced as supportive if it shows an attempt on your part really to try to understand the supervisee's perspective, without adding your interpretation or challenging them to look at it another way. Of course, there is a place for challenging, but here we are focusing on times when your intention is to get across your support for the person.

You can encourage the supervisee by listening particularly for anything which tells you about this person's strengths (e.g. abilities or qualities) in surviving and dealing with the situation, or something that they have achieved or obviously could achieve with the right help. Your summary of this observation can feel especially supportive.

> Pat listens attentively and when Sharma stops and seems to be
> looking to her supervisor for a response, Pat finds herself mute,
> unable to think of anything to say in the face of such a traumatic
> event. However, she pulls herself out of it and suggests that before
> they think about what else could be done, they recap together the
> strengths and achievements that Sharma displayed in dealing with it
> so far, and Pat reflects back some examples: her quick thinking in
> acting appropriately to secure the safety of the patient, the injured
> relative and her colleagues; her resilience in leading her staff through
> what became a long-drawn-out problem.

Tuning in to the emotions which are being expressed or are implicit in what the supervisee is saying can be supportive. To do this, listen particularly to the supervisee's tone, to emotive words or metaphors, so as to imagine yourself in the supervisee's shoes, and to notice the emotional feelings which are stirred up in yourself when you listen. Notice not only which emotions are being expressed or are implicit in what the supervisee is saying, but also the level of intensity of those emotions. You can show that you are tuning in by your non-verbal responses. Occasionally you might say a few words summarising as best you can the emotions and their level of intensity. Put into words and acknowledge the emotion that underlies what the supervisee is saying and its level of intensity, as shown by the cues the supervisee is giving off, e.g. 'So, it seems you are feeling a bit worried about dealing with X?' It's essential to be tentative and allow the supervisee to correct you, to find their own words for their feelings. Your tone needs to be accepting of the emotion, non-critical. This kind of explicit support can be very helpful in enabling the supervisee to develop the central emotional skills of self-awareness and acceptance of their own emotions. For instance, Pat suggests: 'Naturally enough, you seem to be feeling quite shocked and very anxious about this incident. Is that right?'

You can show support by making advocacy statements. By advocacy statements we mean listening to what the supervisee had to say about an experience, and formulating some explicitly supportive responses about this person's rights. While you are listening, you could ask yourself 'Which of the supervisee's individual rights were not respected? What intrusion, humiliation, oppression, deprivation was experienced? What do they deserve as a human being in terms of respect, care, concern, acceptance, protection, information, opportunity, etc.?' Then you could indicate that the supervisee deserves better, perhaps more consideration, information, respect for personal or professional rights, support, etc. For instance, Sharma berates herself for somehow not preventing this incident and she feels a failure for having to involve the police. Pat reminds her that the violent visitor was responsible for his own behaviour and was committing a serious offence and that she and staff and patients had the right to have police protection.

Allowing a supportive silence is essential at times. The supervisee will need space to reflect without interruption or prompting. Allowing emotional release without making a big fuss about it can be supportive. We find that it is not uncommon for nurses to burst into tears with the relief of having protected time and support for themselves, after competently and effectively giving out intensive support to others. Being able to accept this as normal without bleeping the duty psychiatrist is important. The supervisee who can express feelings, release tensions (without taking them out by attacking you), and eventually refocus on reflection and problem solving is emotionally competent. However, this may not be the prevailing attitude in the organisation. The supervisee may berate themselves for expressing feelings or feel embarrassed afterwards. For instance, when Sharma bursts into tears and then struggles to stop them straight away, saying she shouldn't be crying, Pat says: 'You've been through a lot; anyone in your position would need a place to let the tears out and it's OK to do that here'. The supervisee may need some help to recover from releasing feelings. You can gently help them to refocus on the issue or problem at hand, or, if they are too distracted to think straight, to take a mini-break, perhaps making tea or talking about neutral things for a while. For instance, after Sharma has had a good sob and is blowing her nose, and starting to compose herself, Pat asks if she'd like a wet tissue to catch her smeared eye makeup, and damps some tissues in the sink in the corner of the room. Sharma ends up laughing about her makeup and they chat about brands of mascara that are waterproof enough to survive a weep. After a while, Sharma gets back to the topic in question herself and is able to think a little more clearly.

Some self-disclosure on your part can be supportive, when you share a little of your own feelings. For instance, you might explicitly let the supervisee know when you care about them as a person and care about what happens to them. You might share that you also find a certain type of situation difficult. Or that you went through a similar difficulty yourself in the past (this needs to be said with humility, otherwise it may sound patronising). For instance, Pat discloses: 'I felt quite shocked when you told me what you'd been through. I've always found physical violence scary and I admire the way you handled it.'

As the 'pitfalls' sections of this and the next chapter highlight, there is a lot of scope for making mistakes as a clinical supervisor and it can be supportive to admit to it when you have done so and to apologise, without being defensive.

Pitfalls in giving support in clinical supervision

One of the most common pitfalls (see Table 5.3) is to focus prematurely on facts, interrupting the supervisee's flow with factual questions, not letting them explain the situation in their own words and sequence. You rush in with factual questions too quickly. For instance, Sharma is articulate and can describe the situation very well, though her emotional turmoil may have led her to relate the incident a bit out of sequence. Pat would have interrupted and possibly missed the main point if she had fired factual questions such as 'Was he the patient's son or brother?', 'What did you say to him then?', 'Did the visitor lose consciousness after he was knocked down?', 'What did you do next?', 'How long did the police take to arrive?', 'What did the police say were his previous convictions?', 'Who did he attack that time?', 'How long was he in prison before?', and so on. You can avoid this pitfall by mentally tagging any information-seeking questions you want to ask and postponing using them till later. Often you will find that the supervisee covers most of the information you need if they are given space to explain the situation in their own way.

You can avoid this pitfall by reminding yourself that you need to hear the supervisee describe the situation in their own way in order to understand their perception of the situation and their priorities. If you have factual queries, make a mental note to come back to them when the supervisee has finished their explanation.

Similarly, you may prematurely focus on solutions. This is when you jump in with questions which focus on action or when you give advice before the supervisee has had the chance to finish explaining the situation and to reflect upon it in some depth. You can avoid this pitfall by channelling

Table 5.3 Pitfalls in giving support in clinical supervision

- PREMATURE FOCUS ON FACTS OR SOLUTIONS – Interrupting the supervisee's flow with factual questions, not letting them explain the situation in their own words and sequence; focusing on solutions too quickly, interrupting reflection
- LACK OF SUPPORTIVE RESPONSE – No non-verbal response to what the supervisee is saying; lack of explicit verbal support
- ANALYSIS/PARALYSIS – Encouraging supervisee to analyse their feelings, rather than looking at practical ways of dealing with them
- PATRONISING – Talking down to the person as though they are going through a difficult phase that you conquered long ago; speaking in over-simplified manner
- MISPLACED SUPPORT – Colluding, giving encouragement about something you know is not in the supervisee's or their client's best interests
- MOUNTAINS OUT OF MOLEHILLS – Being too earnest, over-dramatising a natural bit of emotional release
- TONE JUDGEMENTAL OR FALSE – Tone comes across as critical, non-accepting or false, using support techniques without genuineness, such as in a back-handed compliment
- TOO DEEP, TOO SOON – You actively delve into supervisee's personal feelings too much (rather than following the supervisee's own pace), thereby increasing vulnerability
- CATHARTIC MANIPULATION – Using techniques which push someone towards releasing feelings
- OVERDONE – Being over the top with compliments which are too general to be useful, or sickly
- ABSORBING STRESS – Taking too much responsibility on yourself for making the supervisee feel better if they are upset; rescuing, trying to take away their emotional discomfort at all costs (but really making yourself feel better), thereby diminishing the person
- OVER-ANALYSIS – You stop the person's emotional flow by asking them to analyse their feelings too soon
- SUPPRESSIVE SYMPATHISING – You overdo the sympathy by swamping them with 'there, theres' or pats on the back

---

your urge to support into making explicit supportive statements, as outlined earlier in this chapter. You could also remind yourself that the purpose of clinical supervision includes in-depth reflection, which requires some patience on your part.

However, there are pitfalls in staying silent too. A deadpan expression, with no non-verbal response to what the supervisee is saying, is inappropriate for a clinical supervisor. The supervisee is likely to feel unnecessarily disconcerted and unsupported. There are schools of psychoanalysis which advocate striving to eliminate personal reactions to the client, to allow for deeper transference to be established, but it is not the role of the clinical supervisor to attract more transference. We have found that some mental health nurses who work with such psychoanalyst colleagues can use the blank approach inappropriately in clinical supervision. In Pat's case, Sharma was looking for something from her and it would have been unnerving to have had a blank response.

Another common pitfall is to assume that by your staying silent, looking at the person and nodding, the supervisee will know that you are listening and supporting. In counselling, the counsellor has more time to show support silently, by their presence and supportive attention during sessions held once, twice or more times a week. The clinical supervisor has less time and needs to be more explicit. The situation that the supervisor talks about may be so traumatic that the supervisee may be mute in response. Saying nothing explicitly supportive may come from inappropriate inhibition: you may not be able to prevent your shock or embarrassment from getting in the way. To avoid this pitfall, try to be aware of your emotions, accept that's how you feel, but go ahead and say something explicitly supportive anyway.

You may miss opportunities to support by trying to get the supervisee to be over-analytical, when you stop the person's emotional flow by asking them to analyse their feelings. Delving into the childhood origins of present-day feelings is the province of counsellors and psychotherapists. The clinical supervisor's focus is on the recent past, the present and the future and your role is to enable expression of emotions and then clarification of how the supervisee can find practical ways of dealing with them, whatever their origins. For instance, if Pat had asked: 'Is feeling responsible for other people's violence a pattern from childhood?', this would have definitely been overstepping the boundaries of clinical supervision.

You might overdo your attempts at explicit support by coming across as patronising. This is easy to do if you are disclosing that you have also had a similar experience, and hint that it was a less mature phase and now you are through it. This can make you sound superior. You can sound patronising if you state the obvious or speak in an over-simplified manner. You might go over the top with compliments which are too general to be useful, such as complimenting the supervisee's personality, rather than their actions. Your tone might sound too sickly. So, keep your support statements low-key and make any reference to your past experience with a tone of humility.

Your support might be misplaced. For instance, by continuing to support the supervisee who is going round in circles, you may be colluding in a blaming state of mind or in avoiding tackling the real problem. You might give encouragement about something you know is not in the supervisee's or their client's best interests, such as a self-destructive course of action. You can avoid this by clarifying what exactly you are supporting and what you are not supporting.

A common pitfall is to make mountains out of molehills by being too earnest and reacting over-dramatically to something that the supervisee can, given time, handle quite well. A supervisee bursting into tears can sometimes trigger this over-reaction from a clinical supervisor, whereas to the supervisee it may be a natural, short-lived bit of emotional release. You can avoid this by looking at your own anxieties when listening to supervisees, accepting that is how you feel and considering ways of containing the anxiety when with your supervisee. This highlights the importance of having your own supervision sessions to deal with such issues.

The clinical supervisor's unaware and uncontained anxiety can lead to an inappropriate tone or manner, perhaps coming across as the opposite of what is intended. For instance, your being tense can result in your sounding judgemental, perhaps your tone coming across as critical, or non-accepting.

Deliberately relaxing your body, especially your throat, can help your tone to come out as you intend. Trying too hard might lead you to sound false, as if you are using support as a technique. A common example is to use a back-handed compliment to soften the blow of criticism; the positive comment has a sting in the tail, ending with a 'but . . .'.

Clinical supervisors who have skills in counselling, mental health nursing or co-counselling may be tempted to use techniques which push someone towards releasing feelings. This may be because you are used to working with people intensively in this area and are using the skills automatically, without considering the different boundaries which should operate in clinical supervision. Sometimes the perspective that 'it will do them good to let it out' makes the clinical supervisor too pushy in this respect. Remembering the following rule of thumb might help here: in clinical supervision, cathartic release of emotions through short periods of crying, storming, shaking and so on are appropriate if the supervisee spontaneously does this or gives definite cues that they wish to do so. Your role is to allow and support this and eventually to help the supervisee to refocus on reflecting on the issues involved. Manipulating or pushing the supervisee into cathartic release is not appropriate: it will only increase their need to protect themselves by resorting to defensive action – and they would be quite right to do so.

Support may be overdone by the clinical supervisor absorbing the supervisee's stress. You take too much responsibility on yourself for making the supervisee feel better if they are upset. You might agree to take action yourself, outside the clinical supervision sessions, rather than enabling supervisees to do it for themselves. You might try to rescue the supervisee from the inevitable emotional discomfort of reflecting on difficult issues. Rescuing comes from the clinical supervisor being unaware of or unable to contain their own feelings of anxiety and helplessness when hearing about the supervisee's difficulties. The suppressive, rescuing behaviour is really to try to make yourself feel better, but diminishes the supervisee. Again, finding ways of becoming more aware and accepting of your own anxieties can pave the way to your being more able to contain them when you are a clinical supervisor. For example, Pat would have been interfering and undermining Sharma if she had offered to facilitate a staff debriefing session on her ward. However, she was aware of the impact that Sharma's clinical supervision session was having on her and knew she could take this to her own clinical supervision. This helped her to contain her anxieties and avoid acting from them inappropriately.

Another pitfall may be over-sympathising, encouraging the supervisee to be repetitively preoccupied with their misery, perhaps swamping them with 'Yes, isn't it awful' comments. This seems especially common in dealing with the despair many nurses feel about the NHS: if this is your feeling too, try not to disappear down the plughole along with your supervisee. Avoid this pitfall by giving some space for expressing feelings, then encouraging the supervisee to move on to reflecting more logically on the issues involved, and practical ways of dealing with the feelings. Use your own supervision to explore emotions that have been triggered by your supervisee.

If you find yourself sliding into one of the pitfalls, all is not lost: you can usually retrieve the situation by recalling that you have many options open to you to show explicit support and choosing the one that feels right.

In summary, the most important principles in supporting the supervisee are:

- giving space, listening and showing that you are listening
- being explicit about your support
- following cues, acknowledging emotions non-judgementally
- using your own supervision for support in dealing with emotions which are stirred up by the supervisee.

The 'being supportive' category needs to be involved in *all* your communication with the supervisee, whether explicitly in your words, or implicitly in your tone and manner.

Catalytic skills of the clinical supervisor

When you use catalytic interventions, you are showing that you are listening and trying to understand, and enabling the supervisee to think aloud, perhaps reflecting on learning from an experience or working through a problem and making their own decision for themselves. In chemistry, a catalyst is a substance which speeds up a chemical reaction without itself becoming part of it. In clinical supervision, using catalytic interventions means you enable the supervisee to reflect in depth on an issue and to move towards clearer learning and decision-making outcomes, without contributing your own perspectives on the issue or solutions.

All the support skills we outlined earlier in this chapter are likely also to have a catalytic function. Often, a supervisee will be able to think more clearly and in more depth from a position of feeling supported. The supervisee who is skilled at using supervision may require little more than support to flourish in her use of the clinical supervision time. However, any supervisee will benefit from the judicious use of some specifically catalytic skills (see Figure 5.3).

When using catalytic skills, you need to have some idea about why you are using them. Although you could say that catalytic methods are comparatively non-directive, in that they do not offer information, advice or challenge, they can often channel the supervisee's thinking in a certain direction. If you use them without due consideration for the reason why you use them, your supervisee may be led up many blind alleys or into scattered thinking, jumping in too many directions. They may end up being more confused than when they started.

Consider four main aims. These would be to enable the supervisee to:

- think aloud and explain the issue in their own words and sequence, given open-ended encouragement
- pick out the most important elements of the issue to explore
- clarify which steps in thinking through an issue they have covered so far
- deepen or move forward in their thinking in focused steps.

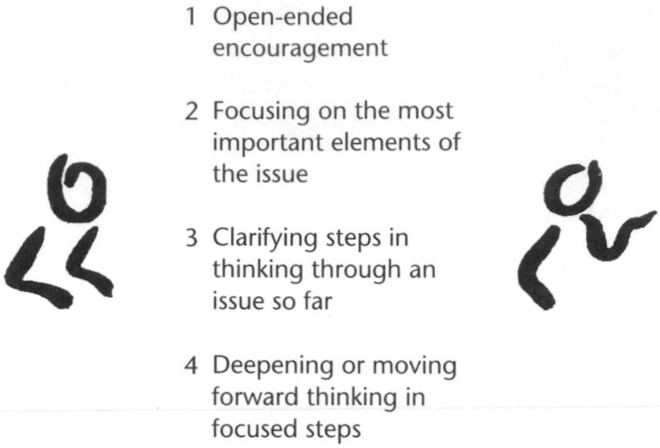

1 Open-ended
  encouragement

2 Focusing on the most
  important elements of
  the issue

3 Clarifying steps in
  thinking through an
  issue so far

4 Deepening or moving
  forward thinking in
  focused steps

Figure 5.3   Steps in using catalytic skills

This framework is an adaptation of Egan's (1975) classic three-stage help-ing framework. The first two aims may be addressed by using support skills and very open catalytic skills, and by allowing or encouraging the supervisee to use the more intuitive methods of reflection suggested in Chapter 3. The last two aims may involve some use of the sequential frameworks for reflec-tion which were suggested in Chapter 4. We do not repeat them again here but encourage you to refer back to them and we especially encourage you to be very selective in the amount of prompts or questions you use to guide the supervisee's thinking: we emphasise the need to follow the supervisee's thinking process as much as possible and add prompts or questions only very infrequently. One well-timed question or prompt may be of much more value than dozens of attempts to control the supervisee's thought processes.

Again, the example of Sharma and Pat will be used to illustrate the skills and pitfalls. In a real clinical supervision session, not all the skills and pitfalls would apply to one session, but here are referred to only as illustrations to bring the text alive.

Open-ended encouragement

All the support skills which were outlined earlier give open-ended encourage-ment to think aloud. Other methods include prompts to continue, last-word echoing and very open questions. Prompts to continue include the many non-verbal encouragements that we give each other in any interaction, such as nods, 'uh huh' 'hm'. Verbal prompts include brief encouragements such as 'yes', 'really?', 'go on', 'and so . . . ?', 'and then . . . ?' You can give a prompt to continue by echoing the last word or phrase, to encourage the super-visee to go on or elaborate (see Table 5.4). Very open questions have little or no specific focus and encourage the supervisee to give more than just a brief reply. Some examples include: 'What would you like to talk about today?', 'What else would you like to say about that?', 'What do you think/ feel about that?'

Table 5.4 Ways of being catalytic in clinical supervision

Open-ended encouragement
- All the support skills outlined earlier
- Prompts to continue: non-verbal encouragement, e.g. nods, 'uh huh', 'hm'; verbal prompts, e.g. 'yes', 'really?', 'go on', 'and so . . . ?', 'and then . . . ?'
- Echoing the last word or phrase
- Very open questions, e.g. 'What would you like to talk about today?', 'What else would you like to say about that?', 'What do you think/feel about that?'

Focusing on the most important elements of the issue
- Selective echoing: echo a significant word or phrase
- Selective summary: pick out the aspects that seem important. Express this tentatively
- Closed questions: questions that could be answered by a brief factual reply or 'yes' or 'no' to help supervisee focus on one aspect
- Invite self-summary: ask supervisee to pick out the main points for themselves
- 'Socratic questioning': encourage the supervisee to imagine that the situation had happened to someone else and they were listening to this other person recounting it. Ask them to imagine what they would want to say to that person

Clarifying steps in thinking through an issue so far
- 'Learning from experience cycle' diagnosis: spot the stages the supervisee has covered in her thinking so far and give feedback on this using one of the reflective cycle models
- Problem-solving diagnosis: spot the stages that the supervisee has covered in one of the problem-solving models

Deepening or moving forward thinking in focused steps
- Revisit a previous stage in one of the reflective or problem-solving models
- Deepen their exploration of the stage they have reached
- Emotional barometer: noticing own strong feelings and using this awareness to enable the supervisee to acknowledge her own emotional feelings
- Logical building: summarise the content of what the supervisee is saying and point to any direction in which it seems to be leading
- Focus open questions on the next step in the cycle

Focusing on the most important elements of the issue

You could use selective echoing, selective summary, closed questions, inviting self-summary and 'Socratic questioning' to help the supervisee to focus on the most important aspects of the issue being discussed.

Selective echoing is when you echo a specific word or phrase that seems especially significant, in order to encourage the supervisee to explore a bit further.

> Sharma: 'It was like I was watching myself dealing with it, I couldn't believe my hands were so steady. . . . (pause)'.
> Pat: 'Couldn't believe it?'

Any summary you make of what the supervisee is saying will have an element of selection about it: you will automatically pick out the aspects that have had an impact on you, that seem important. It is important to be aware of this and to be tentative in offering the summary: you may have missed the most important point as far as the supervisee is concerned. You can express this tentativeness by adding a checking-out question or by making your settlement sound like a question.

'So far, you seem to be saying . . . Have I missed out anything important?' 'Do you mean that you . . . ?' 'It seems to me that the most immediately important aspect of this situation is . . . ?'

Closed questions are questions that could be answered by a brief factual reply or 'yes' or 'no', and are useful to help the supervisee focus on one aspect.

Pat: 'Is it that in spite of acting professionally, inside you felt in a state of shock?'

You could invite a self-summary by asking the supervisee to reflect back over what they have said and to pick out the main points for themselves.

Pat: 'Looking back over what you've told me so far about this very difficult situation, what would you like to focus on in particular in the time we have left here together?'

One way of helping the supervisee to step back and pick out what is important is by using 'Socratic questioning': you encourage the supervisee to imagine that the situation had happened to someone else and they were listening to this other person recounting it.

Pat: 'You've already said you can step back and observe yourself while you were dealing with all this: let's take that a bit further. Imagine that the time is now two weeks ago, before this happened. A colleague, let's call her Abigail, comes to you and tells you exactly what you've told me, about how she had to deal with a relative (with a history of convictions for grievous bodily harm) of a semi-comatose, dying patient who had been physically violent with another relative and verbally violent and threatening towards staff. What would you think about Abigail and her situation?'

Clarifying steps in thinking so far

The supervisee may be intuitively or consciously using elements of some of the reflective frameworks outlined in Chapter 4. Whilst you are listening you may be able to spot the stages the supervisee has covered in her thinking so far and give feedback to clarify this. Whilst each of the frameworks we offered focused on specific lines of thought, the supervisee may not follow only one framework but may have covered elements of two or more of them.

For instance, Pat sees the stages that Sharma has gone through in the 'learning from experience' spiral outlined in Chapter 4 and in Figure 4.7. She has described the experience in terms of the events and her observations of her own and other people's actions and reactions, and looked in some depth at her feelings about the issue. She is in some confusion about the meaning of it all and is jumping towards evaluating her performance in a negative, self-blaming way. Pat shares these observations with Sharma before going on to encouraging her to analyse the meaning of the situation in more depth.

You might find it useful to make a problem-solving diagnosis: you spot the stages that the supervisee has covered in one of the problem-solving frameworks. Again, these were outlined in Chapter 4.

For instance, Pat recognises that Sharma has done some excellent on-the-spot problem solving and is now preoccupied with the last stage of the problem-solving spiral suggested in Chapter 4, Figure 4.4: 'So, you seem to be struggling to find something else to be done, some other action to take, when it seems to me you have covered every angle and there's nothing else practical to be done at this point. Is that so?'

Deepening or moving forward thinking in focused steps

Having clarified to yourself and possibly to the supervisee where they seem to be in their thinking, you might help the supervisee either to revisit a previous stage in one of the reflective or problem-solving frameworks, or to deepen their exploration of the stage they have reached or to move on to the next step. As far as possible, without interrupting the supervisee's flow, try to be transparent about which framework you are using. This may help the supervisee to understand the reflective framework and be able to use it more in everyday practice.

For example, Pat sees that Sharma might usefully go back to the beginning of the problem-solving cycle and redefine the present problem: 'I'm wondering if it would be useful to focus on what the main difficulty is for you right now?' Sharma seems confused and repeats some of the information she has shared previously. Pat makes a quick drawing of the problem-solving cycle to remind Sharma of a framework they have discussed in the past.

You may be able to enable the supervisee to identify unacknowledged emotions by using yourself as an emotional barometer. At times, you may find that you have a strong emotional reaction to what the supervisee is saying or to her manner. It is possible that as the clinical supervisor you pick up the supervisee's unacknowledged strength of feeling. Helping the supervisee to acknowledge and accept her emotions can be an important step in deepening her reflection and enable her to move on. This 'emotional barometer' phenomenon (described as counter-transference in Chapter 2) can extend as far as the client: the client has unacknowledged feelings which become stirred up in the supervisee; the supervisee does not acknowledge them in herself and the clinical supervisor then feels them too. Enabling the supervisee to acknowledge her feelings can in turn help her to enable the client to acknowledge hers.

You need to be tentative in using this catalytic method: bear in mind the 'fifty-fifty benchmark': that 50 per cent of the time your strong feeling reactions to the supervisee reflect the supervisee's unacknowledged feelings; and 50 per cent of the time the feelings are nothing to do with the supervisee at all, but relate only to your own past experiences. Even if you are right, the supervisee may not be ready to explore those feelings and anything other than a tentative approach on your part can be too intrusive and cross the boundaries between clinical supervision and psychotherapy.

As an example of using the 'emotional barometer': when Pat was first listening to Sharma describing the situation, she noticed that she herself felt shocked and for a while did not know what to do or say. She tentatively uses this to help Sharma become more aware of the emotional factor. Pat: 'Is it that the main difficulty at the moment for yourself and your team is in experiencing delayed shock and traumatic feelings and now that everything practical has been attended to you're at a loss as to what to do?' This hits the spot and Sharma talks for some time about her own feelings and her concern for her team members, and Pat uses occasional supportive statements.

The supervisee will often herself be moving forward in her thinking without realising it. 'Logical building' is a way of enabling her to clarify this: you summarise the content of what the supervisee is saying and point to any direction in which it seems to be leading. For example, after some time, Pat summarises where Sharma seems to have got to in the 'Emotional learning' framework outlined in Chapter 4 (Figure 4.11, p. 122) and suggests a way forward: 'It seems you're very aware of your own emotional reactions and those of your colleagues and have come to some acceptance of these as being normal human reactions to this situation and have been dealing with them by redirecting the energy into appropriate practical action. Now that there is nothing else practical to do, I wonder what other ways you could now express and contain the feelings that are likely to keep welling up?' Sharma begins to think about the possibility that she can meet with other ward manager colleagues and ask for support time and that she can build in emotional debriefing sessions with her team. Pat uses 'logical building' again: 'So, you've decided to see about getting more support time for yourself. What's your first step in getting this arranged?' And then later on: 'You also decided to have debriefing sessions for your staff. How will you go about that exactly?'

Pitfalls in using catalytic skills

One of the most common pitfalls (see also Table 5.5) is interrogating: when you machine gun the supervisee with questions or prompts, going through your own checklist rather than giving the supervisee the chance to explain in her own words. This links to the first of the pitfalls in supporting. You may become prematurely action-oriented, coming in with advice about solutions or inviting the supervisee to plan what they are going to do before they have reflected more deeply on the issue. You would be encouraging shallow thinking by doing this and perhaps insulting the supervisee's intelligence by covering options she had already considered or dealt with. In Sharma's case, she had dealt conscientiously with all practical aspects of the situation and Pat would have demeaned her by coming in with action-oriented advice before Sharma had a chance to tell the whole story. One way to avoid this pitfall is to remember the frameworks for reflection and problem solving and remind yourself that your role is to enable in-depth reflection, not instant advice-giving.

On the other hand, over-processing results from being too attached to one of the frameworks for reflection or problem solving. In this case you have one fixed framework in mind and relentlessly question the supervisee to hound them to think sequentially through the framework. These frameworks should be used as mere tools to pick up and put down when needed. Most supervisees will move between frameworks or back and forth between stages of one framework rather than follow a pre-programmed thought pathway. One way to avoid over-processing is to be sure that you have enough understanding of more than one framework for reflection and for problem solving and to use a mixture in your own reflection during your own clinical supervision. This will help you to be able to stand back and observe which elements of which frameworks the supervisee is using and summarise and validate what thinking she has done herself.

Answering your own questions can be a pitfall. This is when you follow an open question with a closed one which indicates your answer. For instance: Pat: 'What do you think about your staff nurse's reactions? Don't you think she has a right to feel upset?' If this is one of your tendencies, imagine a large full stop hanging in the air after you have asked an open question. Give the supervisee time to pause and reply in her own time. 'Don't you think she has a right to feel upset?' is also an example of a leading question. Leading questions are a common pitfall: these are questions phrased in a way which indicates what answer you expect the supervisee to give.

Another common pitfall is curiosity-questioning. This is when you ask questions to satisfy your own interest and curiosity. This can lead the supervisee off on a tangent, away from the issue that is most concerning her at this time. Some of the examples under 'interrogating' could be curiosity-led questions. One way of avoiding this pitfall is to stop yourself by thinking 'This is *her* time' and focusing back on what the supervisee is saying.

Following the red herring may be a diversion as a result of your directing the topic towards your focus of interest, but can also be a result of the supervisee diverting away from an uncomfortable issue onto something more comfortable but less relevant which diverts from the decision to be made.

Over-confident use of the 'emotional barometer' might lead you to being pushy about what the supervisee *ought* to be feeling, when you may be mistaken about the emotional issues. Your reading of the emotional issues involved may be more about you and your past experiences than about the supervisee's present feeling state.

Being compulsively catalytic can be a pitfall for someone who is a recent convert to non-directive approaches to facilitating reflection in clinical supervision. There will be times when giving advice or information would be more appropriate than relentlessly putting everything back to the supervisee to work out or find out for themselves. For instance, Pat may have information about a helpful pamphlet outlining a suggested process for debriefing after traumatic situations that has been produced by staff at the psychiatric hospital that is part of the same Trust and it would be more helpful for her to give Sharma a copy than to struggle on without it.

Heron (1990: 155) highlights some pitfalls to bear in mind: 'dull antenna', 'interview rape', 'scraping the bowl', 'compulsive search for order'

Table 5.5   Pitfalls in being catalytic in clinical supervision

---

- INTERROGATING – Machine gunning the supervisee with factual questions
- PREMATURELY ACTION-ORIENTED – Advice about solutions or inviting the supervisee to plan what they are going to do before they have reflected more deeply on the issue
- OVER-PROCESSING – Being too attached to one of the models for reflection or problem solving and relentlessly questioning the supervisee to hound them to think sequentially through the model
- ANSWERING YOUR OWN QUESTIONS – Following an open question with a closed one which indicates your answer
- CURIOSITY-QUESTIONING – Questions to satisfy your own interest and curiosity may lead the supervisee off on a tangent, away from the issue that is most concerning her at this time
- FOLLOWING THE RED HERRING – Diversion as a result of your directing the topic towards your focus of interest, but can also be as a result of the supervisee diverting away from an uncomfortable issue onto something more comfortable but less relevant
- COMPULSIVELY CATALYTIC – Relentlessly putting everything back to the supervisee to work out or find out for themselves rather than giving advice or information appropriately
- DULL ANTENNA – Miss important cues and instead blunder on to something less important to the supervisee
- INTERVIEW RAPE – Probe into private aspects of the person's life or feelings without invitation
- PUSHY USE OF EMOTIONAL BAROMETER – over-determined use of this method
- SCRAPING THE BOWL – Going over ground which supervisee has discussed, decided and finished with
- COMPULSIVE SEARCH FOR ORDER – Push supervisee into being more coherent than they are ready to be
- PREMATURE CLOSURE – Pushing the supervisee to reach a neat conclusion to reflecting on a topic so you yourself have a sense of completion

---

and 'premature closure'. 'Dull antenna' is when you miss important cues and instead blunder on to something less important to the supervisee. For example, if Pat had pursued the topic of the violent man's past history, she might have missed the important issue, which was the state of shock and trauma that Sharma and her team were experiencing.

'Interview rape' is when you probe into private aspects of the person's life or feelings without invitation. In Pat's case, she did not fall into this pitfall in opening up the emotional area: she followed Sharma's cues into the issue of shock. If she had asked 'How is all this strain affecting your home life, your relationship with your partner?', she would have been veering towards 'interview rape': she is attempting to open up a private topic when she has had no cues or invitation to do so.

'Scraping the bowl' involves going over ground which the supervisee has discussed, decided and finished with. 'Compulsive search for order' is when you try to push the supervisee into being more coherent than they are ready to be. For instance, Sharma needed to blurt out the story to Pat, and did it in a fairly illogical way, getting the sequence out of order. If Pat had interrupted and demanded that she get her thoughts more organised in the early stages of the session, she would have been falling into this pitfall.

'Premature closure' is pushing the supervisee to reach a neat conclusion to reflecting on a topic so you yourself have a sense of completion. Working in a facilitative role such as clinical supervisor can leave you with some frustration when the supervisee does not achieve a neat solution or plan by the end of the discussion. This frustration goes with the role and you will need to learn to sit with it. The supervisee is capable of continuing to reflect on the issue after the session, without your help, and may need some more time or information in order to come to an appropriate conclusion.

The focus in this chapter has been on the clinical supervisor but this must be placed in the context of the working alliance between supervisee and clinical supervisor. Effective use of these skills requires an underlying care and concern for the supervisee and her client/patients and a desire to see them flourish. Any tendency to want to use a slick array of techniques needs to be privately acknowledged and contained, otherwise the supervisee will sense a lack of genuineness and respect. You may have to modify your own defensive reactions, and be alert to any tendency towards being over-critical or a desire to take over and dazzle with your own experience. Bear in mind that the purpose of support and catalytic skills is to provide a secure enough psychological base within which the supervisee can feel supported enough to take on the challenge of learning and developing their clinical practice, and their part in the complexity and quality of that practice that they play as a person. The opportunity that the supervisee gets in thinking these issues through for herself builds the skill of the 'internal supervisor' that will be used in everyday practice.

The next chapter examines the more authoritative skills used occasionally by the clinical supervisor.

Informative and challenging skills of the clinical supervisor

6

Most of the help that you as clinical supervisor give to the supervisee is in the form of support and catalytic facilitation of the supervisee's own reflection on issues affecting practice. You will usually need to be very sparing in giving information, advice or challenging, but this authoritative dimension of the role of the clinical supervisor or supervision group member is an essential element of the process. In Chapter 2 we asked you to think about the use of power within the clinical supervision relationship, and suggested that there was a great deal of confusion and ambivalence about its use in all professional relationships, both with clients and colleagues. On the one hand, nurses can often have a tendency to give too much information and advice: this is shown in numerous communication studies in nursing (see the literature review in Kendall 1991). On the other, there is a tendency to avoid using challenging, illustrated by Burnard and Morrison's study (1988). Although the clinical supervisor's repertoire of non-directive skills is crucial for encouraging a working alliance, centring on professional growth and support, clinical supervisors need to balance this with more directive approaches. We find that once nurses learn the effectiveness of support and catalytic skills, they can sometimes become excessively non-directive, withholding information, advice or challenge inappropriately as far as the clinical supervision relationship is concerned. In Chapter 2 we suggested that some practitioners shy away from or minimise the authoritative dimension of their role and can be quick to feel anxious or resistant to perceived authority themselves and in others. In this chapter you are urged to remember the distinction we drew in Chapter 2 between authoritative and authoritarian, when we suggested that authoritative skills were based on valid experience, knowledge and skills, which can be used non-abusively to enable and support others.

This chapter will focus on the skills necessary to achieve an appropriately authoritative approach. This is consistent with the concern nurses have about professional accountability *and* standards and with the support and growth principles of clinical supervision. Our examples focus on directive skills in the 'average' clinical supervision session, which is what we have observed, rather than the catastrophic 'what if' examples that come to mind when we first begin to discuss this dimension with nurses. The skills are the focus of this chapter and can be applied to whatever level of concern, although their use is also often brought into sharp relief when there is specific concern about accountability and standards.

Informative skills

We distinguish between giving information and giving advice in that giving information is sharing facts, opinions, procedures in order that the supervisee can extrapolate and make her own informed decision about what course of action to take. Giving advice is offering one or more examples of specific courses of action that the supervisee herself can take when considering her options. Again, the emphasis is on the supervisee making the decision about what action to take: she remains responsible for her practice whatever advice you give as clinical supervisor. We encourage you to give any information, advice, instructions in such a way that the supervisee can take it or leave it, use it in their decision making or not, and, if you have a tendency to be too informative, to restrain yourself in using this skill and focus on developing the other three skills more.

Giving information or advice, rather than purely support and catalytic help, is appropriate when certain conditions apply. A general rule of thumb is that the more technical a problem is, the more relevant it is to offer information or advice. The more the issue concerns feelings and human relationships (the most common issues that we see brought to clinical supervision), the less appropriate it is to be informative. However, it may be appropriate in the following scenarios:

- the supervisee is stuck in their thinking; support and catalytic help has not worked, so some information or advice about intuitive methods of reflection or frameworks for problem solving or reflection may unblock her (see Chapter 4)
- the supervisee is going along the wrong track because they are genuinely unaware of or do not understand some key facts or options that would easily clarify the situation
- the supervisee's gaps in knowledge, misunderstanding, misinformation, are a part of the problem that they bring to clinical supervision or are likely to experience soon
- the supervisee is floundering because their confidence and decision-making ability is shattered and some key information or advice would start them on the road to doing something to rectify a situation and begin to get their confidence back
- the supervisee is totally unaware of some important information or options and you need to share these in order to help the supervisee to progress and make informed decisions and choices about what to do

- the situation is critical and requires quick action
- the problem is within your specialist field of expertise and the supervisee knows little about it
- the supervisee has asked for information or advice and giving it would not be colluding with inappropriate dependency on the clinical supervisor
- the supervisee has decided to take precipitate action which has not been thought through and is obviously inappropriate, too risky for herself or others or is an incorrect procedure, and strong advice is required to help her get back on track
- the supervisee seems to be stuck in a cycle of behaviour which is destructive and attempts to help supportively and with catalytic and challenging interventions have not worked, so repeated firm advice is necessary.

Two examples will be used in this section:

Marie is a staff nurse on an accident and emergency unit, attending a clinical supervision session with her staff nurse colleague Toby (they use a circular arrangement of peer supervision, shown in Chapter 8, Table 8.6). She is reflecting on a problem with confronting a student nurse about her attitude towards patients, not being willing to share information to allow them to take part in making their own decisions about treatment. In passing, she mentions that she was about to show the student how to treat a patient with hypothermia with a space blanket, but couldn't find one. She asks Toby if he happens to know where they are kept nowadays, since it has been years since a patient with hypothermia has been admitted while she's been on duty.

Kunu is a member of a clinical supervision group and is attending a session which happens to be held on the last day of her annual leave, but she has come into work just for the session. She was about to use her time in the clinical supervision session to talk through some long-term plans for managing the team on her unit that she had thought through while on holiday in West Africa. She was unaware that there had been plans made at Trust board level which would affect her unit, and Laura felt she had to let her have the information now.

Steps in giving information

You may have a vast amount of information on a topic but the supervisee is likely only to require a small amount of it. Assessing which specific aspects of the topic is required is important, otherwise you will swamp the supervisee with information or enthusiasm (see Figure 6.1). First of all find out what the supervisee exactly wants or needs to know. Then find out the supervisee's existing level of knowledge, what the supervisee already knows about the topic. You will be using your catalytic skills to elicit this information: for instance: 'What exactly would you like to know about . . . ?', 'Tell me what you know already about . . . ?', 'Have you ever tried to do this or seen anyone doing this before?'

Toby checks with Marie: 'You don't remember the change of procedure?' Laura checks by asking: 'Kunu, before you go on, am I right in thinking you don't start back till tomorrow, you haven't been to the ward yet? . . . So you haven't heard the bad news?'

Then give the information in small steps: give a little information at a time and try to relate it to the supervisee's situation or to her choice of words. Leave space for questions and, after each step, check for understanding before going on to the next step. Be careful to stop yourself when you have given enough and give the supervisee time to mull it over. It can be useful to make notes or a diagram of the main points and give it to the supervisee to keep, since about 70 per cent of verbally-given information is forgotten in a short time if there is no written or visual backup to reinforce it.

Toby: 'We don't use space blankets any more, they've been proved to be OK for prevention but by the time people get to us with definite hypothermia, they're not effective enough.' Marie says: 'Well, that one passed me by. Maybe it's because I've been taking my annual leave in the winter the last few years, when it was all happening. What are we supposed to do now?' Toby: 'Can you remember what we did before we had space blankets?' Marie: 'Yes, we just had to rely on warming everything, blankets, oxygen, IVs and so on.' Toby: 'That's it, you've got it, we're back to that, the studies have shown it's more effective. I'll bring you some references next time if you like. Anyway, you were saying about this student nurse's attitude?' Laura: 'I'm sorry to have to tell you this. Your manager was probably going to meet you tomorrow to tell you. As far as I understand it, the plan is to close your ward and Nightingale ward in four weeks' time.'

Checking for understanding involves using your catalytic skills again: use open questions such as 'What has struck you in particular about what I've just said?', 'Which parts of that are especially relevant to your situation?', 'How might you use this information?' Closed questions like 'OK?', 'Is that clear?', 'Did you understand?', or 'Got that?' are not going to give you a good idea of what the supervisee has really understood.

Toby checked Marie's understanding by asking her to recap on her existing knowledge and then confirmed it. In Kunu's case, there was no need to check: she understood only too well. After phoning her manager to get confirmation she rejoined the group in a state of shock and spent the session getting support from them.

Ways of giving advice

Advice-giving is distinguished from information-giving in that advice is a suggestion for action. There are two types of advice: soft and firm advice.

Soft advice is appropriate for most clinical supervision situations. You give the advice as one suggestion or option, implying or explicitly pointing out

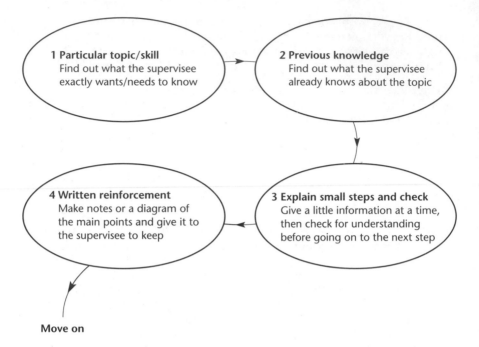

Figure 6.1 Steps in giving information

that there are other courses of action that might be equally effective. You phrase the advice tentatively, for instance: 'I suggest . . .', 'You could try . . .', 'You might . . .', 'Possibly . . .', 'One thing you could try is . . .', 'One option could be . . .' and so on.

You would give firm advice when you feel strongly about the course of action you are suggesting. You still need to be conscious that the supervisee has the right to reject your advice, but that they must take responsibility for the consequences of doing so. Express your strength of conviction and spell out the consequences of not following the advice: for instance: 'I strongly advise/urge/suggest you do such and such, otherwise — will probably happen', 'It's vital/very important/essential that you — or else — will happen'.

In giving advice, it is preferable to be positive: to speak more of 'dos' rather than 'don'ts'. Of course, you may need to point out pitfalls but emphasise the positive course of action that you are suggesting the supervisee takes. Someone who is stressed or confused may be more confused or get the wrong end of the stick if you emphasise the 'don'ts'. You can see this when, say, helping a very disorientated patient to eat: if you say 'Don't spit this out' the patient often does just what you said, not registering the 'Don't'. 'Try to chew this and swallow it' usually gets a better response. Likewise a stressed supervisee: say what you positively advise the supervisee to do, not what you don't want them to do. Giving a positive instruction puts the positive idea in the other person's mind and reduces misunderstanding.

Pitfalls in being informative

The most common pitfall we have seen is swamping the supervisee with too much information, advice or enthusiasm for the subject, so the supervisee has no space to mull over and apply relevant information. Consciously stopping, allowing pauses and checking for understanding can help you to slow down and avoid getting carried away. We find that the nurses who have a tendency to give too much information or advice may do so as a means of showing they want to explicitly support the supervisee. In this case, learning about the skills of giving explicit support, as shown in the previous chapter, can reduce this tendency.

Related to this is giving information or advice which is not wanted: perhaps the supervisee knows already, or is quite capable of working it out for themselves, or is giving off cues that they do not want it at that point. An extreme version of this is interfering: giving information or advice about problems which are nothing to do with your expertise or your contract with the supervisee. You can avoid this pitfall by checking if some advice or information is wanted before you give it. Here you need to be sensitive to cues of hesitancy or uncertainty: nurses will often not find it easy to say no. It may be important to you as a clinical supervisor to be seen as someone who has something to offer, to be identified as the knowledgeable person who solved a difficult situation. Coping with your feelings of lack of acknowledgement and appreciation are part of the job: the more effective you are at facilitating, the more the supervisee will be pleased with herself for solving the problem, rather than pleased with you. The origins of giving too much advice may lie in a need to help by rescuing the supervisee from the discomfort of puzzling something through for herself: the clinical supervisor cannot bear her own discomfort while sitting with the supervisee. However, whatever the motives, Casement (1985) reminds us to stay with not-knowing, when the issue is one of feelings or human relationships: anything else can be either too premature or too dishonest.

You might become too attached to your advice, perhaps being over-anxious about it being taken, hounding the supervisee with reminders and follow-ups. Even though other options may be equally or more effective you may show annoyance that the supervisee hasn't taken your excellent advice.

Your manner can come across as a put-down if your tone implies that the supervisee is stupid for not knowing the information or not knowing what to do. This can happen when you feel surprised that the supervisee appears not to know something basic or cannot see the obvious solution to the problem. Avoid this pitfall by remembering that stress can make the supervisee forget or temporarily be blind to the obvious, and that this probably happens to you sometimes too. Remember also that you do not know every single detail of the supervisee's story: there may be other factors that get in the way of the obvious solutions that are unknown to you but known to the supervisee.

The clinical supervision can come across as patronising if giving information which the supervisee already knows well. Also, if you have had a similar experience but the way you share it implies that you are now more mature, through that phase now, this can sound patronising. Likewise using over-simplified vocabulary or showing exaggerated patience by using a sing-song, nursery teacher tone of voice. Finding out what the supervisee already knows, or helping them to remember and have confidence in their own know-ledge, can help avoid this pitfall.

The delivery of information or advice may be ineffective: too fast, slow, indistinct, too enthusiastic, too flat or boring, with no written reinforcement or too complicated, using terms not known by the supervisee. Following the guidelines suggested earlier may avoid this pitfall, especially eliciting the supervisee's specific wants and needs and their previous knowledge. You can then use some of the supervisee's vocabulary in your explanation, and relate your points to their concerns.

'Compulsive counselling' may occur when the clinical supervisor con-tinues to use support and catalytic interventions when some information or advice may be more appropriate. This seems to happen most often with nurses who are used to listening non-directively to clients for long periods of time, such as mental health nurses or nurses with a specific counselling role. Alternatively, a clinical supervisor who is a fervent recent convert to non-directive approaches may have a tendency to overdo non-direction.

Challenging skills

Your intention in challenging the supervisee is to help them to be more aware of behaviour or values which actually or potentially contribute to the problem in question, or which block their potential for developing high quality practice, or block their ability to use clinical supervision well.

Most people on clinical supervision courses find this skill is one of their weakest. The exceptions seem to be those whose work involves the necessity for using challenging skills a lot, such as those who work in substance abuse clinics, secure units and accident and emergency departments. Burnard and Morrison (1988) also found that nurses found challenging to be the most stressful and difficult interpersonal skill to use. It causes anxiety for almost everyone, partly because in reality you never really know how the supervisee will react and partly because of the emotional baggage we bring from our own past experiences of being on the receiving end of destructive criticism. You may not wish to upset the supervisee, but, as Egan (1975) points out, people have enough emotional resilience to be able to manage the dis-comfort that can result from having behaviour and values challenged in a supportive way.

Historically there has been very little help for practitioners to learn and practise challenging skills. This framework will help to focus on ways of following through your intention to challenge, but probably nothing will completely take away the inevitable anxiety of challenging. However, the principles and step-by-step format offered here may help you to manage that anxiety.

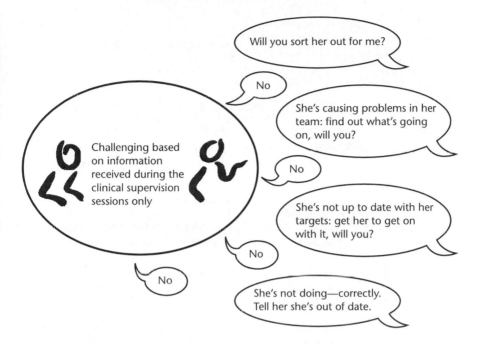

Figure 6.2 Keeping your challenging within the boundaries of the clinical supervision relationship

Some conditions for challenging the supervisee

As a clinical supervisor, you have the right and responsibility to challenge issues that concern or alarm you, *provided that you have gained the information during the clinical supervision sessions* (see Figure 6.2). This means that if you see or discover errors elsewhere, outside the sessions, it is important that you challenge them there and then rather than comment during the clinical supervision session. It also means that if someone else asks you to challenge the supervisee about something they are concerned about, it is important that you refuse and put it back to them to deal with. Otherwise you undermine the principles of clinical supervision, collude with whoever is abdicating their responsibility and you also undermine their authority. This type of request is often reported by clinical supervisors attending our courses.

The second condition is that the supervisee does not appear to have insight into the negative effect of their behaviour or values, chooses to ignore it or does not take it seriously enough. Third, you have already used supportive and catalytic facilitation and these have not succeeded in raising awareness. Alternatively, the issue is of such pressing importance that it would be inappropriate to spend time using these other approaches.

Bear in mind that the supervisee has enough emotional resilience to be able to manage the discomfort that can result from having gaps in knowledge or ability exposed and from having behaviour and values challenged.

Topics for challenging the supervisee

You need to be clear about what it is exactly that you are challenging about what the person does.

Mistakes

You might need to challenge the supervisee about specific mistakes, whether errors in clinical procedures that the supervisee is recounting, a judgement that you consider is mistaken or perhaps dealing with the interpersonal aspects of the problem under discussion in what you consider to be an inappropriate manner.

> Jacky is describing to Blossom a complicated interaction between herself, a patient and a doctor, which happened while she and the doctor were helping the patient to turn over in bed. The patient was recovering from a total hip replacement. She mentions in passing that they had not bothered to use an Immuturn frame.

Broken contracts

The supervisee might be describing an event in which she appears not to have fulfilled a contract, whether with her client, team members or employers. This might be an explicit organisational contract, such as working a certain number of hours or carrying out certain functions or may be an explicit person-to-person agreement between the supervisee and a client or colleague. Implicit contracts are more about what people might reasonably expect from each other according to their roles.

> Barbara is telling her clinical supervisor Pauline about a conflict with her new manager. Pauline has always refused to sort out the holiday roster directly with her two immediate health visitor colleagues, with whom she is barely on speaking terms. The previous manager used to do it for them to keep the peace.

Not working to the UKCC (1992a) Code of Professional Conduct

There may be aspects of the *Code of Professional Conduct* which the supervisee appears not to be working to, and clear or more subtle gaps in the practice of their accountability.

> David tells his clinical supervisor Hannah about having witnessed a colleague repeatedly slapping a patient with learning difficulties. David has reported this verbally to the team leader who has done nothing about it, apparently not believing him and pathologising his concern, by saying that David is having a very difficult time due to a marriage break-up and needs support: the abuse continues. He feels that he has fulfilled his responsibilities, considers that no further action is required on his part and washes his hands of the affair.

Mental blocks

These are the defences, mental rigidities or emotional blind spots which get in the supervisee's own way.

Carol has spoken to her clinical supervisor Zara about a difficulty with a colleague who is not pulling her weight in the team. At the last two clinical supervision sessions she has gone away with an action plan to confront the colleague but keeps procrastinating.

Misuse of clinical supervision time
Clinical supervisors often report that supervisees have difficulties in the early stages of clinical supervision with taking responsibility for their use of the time in clinical supervision. This is especially the case if the supervisee has not been able to attend training in supervisee skills, or has chosen not to attend such courses on offer. Lack of understanding of clinical supervision, lack of skill in reflection or resentment about having to attend may contribute to this type of situation.

Rob tends to describe a problem to his clinical supervisor Mohammed in a manner that implies: 'There it is, now see if you can sort it out'.

Inconsistencies
There may be a lack of fit between what the supervisee thinks she does and what she actually does. The inconsistency may be between the supervisee's espoused values and her behaviour.

Danielle is complaining to Pete about an agency nurse who is temporarily in her team and seems to be slow in learning the ropes. She recounts some of their conversations in which it sounds as if Danielle has frequently been quite harsh and the agency nurse goes to pieces when she is on duty, but apparently not when Danielle's deputy is in charge. Danielle maintains she is always patient with new staff but that this person is beyond the pale and she is thinking of contacting the agency to get her replaced.

Signs of an unacknowledged problem
The supervisee may be talking negatively about her patients/clients or her colleagues in such a way that you sense there is some underlying problem which has not been acknowledged.

Fran notices that Roxanne (a nursery nurse) is complaining a lot about the parents of the patients she works with on the paediatric ward.

Prejudices and unfounded assumptions
The supervisee may exhibit some negative assumptions about certain sectors of society, such as people of a different race, class, religion, sexuality, age, level of physical or mental ability and so on. She may make unfounded assumptions about people who are different from herself.

Marjorie is a practice nurse and describes to her clinical supervisor Norma how she enjoys working at the main surgery premises, her practice base, but dislikes holding clinics in the satellite surgery situated in a large housing estate. She speaks of the residents of the estate as 'riff-raff'.

Challenging: some principles

Focus on positive change: the challenge should be given in the spirit that
the supervisee has the potential for positive change and that your role is to
help them towards that. Your tone therefore should avoid sounding punitive. (See Figure 6.3.)

It is very important that you comment only on the supervisee's actions,
decisions or apparent values, *not* on their personality. Commenting on personality will feel more like a personal attack and is not supportive of change
since the supervisee cannot do anything immediately tangible to change
their personality, even if they wanted to.

Be supportive. When you have challenged a supervisee, be prepared to let
them respond and have their say: that in itself is supportive. You may wish
to draw them out about any background reasons or feelings about the problem, or to offer other support. The manner in which you say the challenge
needs to be supportive rather than carping or critical. Remember, your intention is to raise awareness and throw some light on the situation, not to
punish or take out your frustrations on the supervisee. Ensure that you offer
support towards change, such as encouraging the supervisee to explore the
issue further and consider other approaches that might be more positive.

Comment on issues arising during the clinical supervision session only.

Be specific: it is important that you refer to specific actions or things
the supervisee has said to you. Avoid generalities, such as 'You always . . .'.

Speak concisely: you may not need to say it all at once, so be brief. Allow
silences so the supervisee can absorb and respond. The inevitable anxiety
involved in challenging tends to lead many people to say too much or repeat
themselves, not allowing the supervisee the space to have her say.

Challenging questions
These are focused on enabling the supervisee to think through what they
have said and come to some insight about the issue at hand.

> Pete to Danielle: 'You say you are always patient with new staff.
> In what ways have you been patient with this agency nurse?'

> Hannah to David: 'Do you really think that your responsibilities
> end there?'

Challenging statements
At times, it might be clearer to get to the point and make a challenging
statement rather than ask a question. The steps shown in the 'Challenging'
map (Figure 6.3) can help to make the challenging statement constructive.
You will be selecting and using elements of this map in the order that is
appropriate to the situation.

Sometimes you may need to pinpoint the topic upon which you want to
comment, especially if the discussion has gone off the point towards something else.

> Norma: 'I'd like to say something about the way you referred earlier
> to the residents of the estate'.

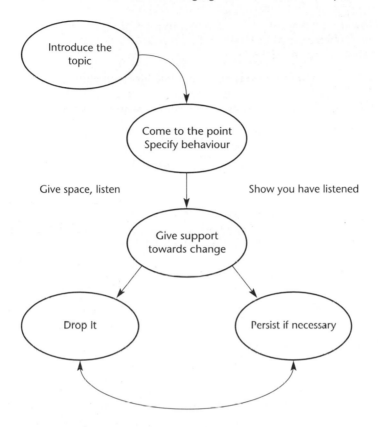

Give space, listen

Show you have listened

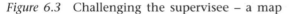

Figure 6.3 Challenging the supervisee – a map

Come to the point as quickly and concisely as possible and explain how the person falls short. Speak in the first person: for example, 'I'm concerned that you called them "riff-raff". I don't think this attitude is acceptable.'

Let the supervisee react in their own time. People have different ways of reacting to the discomfort of being challenged and need time to respond. Listen carefully to what they say and show that you have listened by referring to what they have said. A challenge is more likely to escalate into an argument if the supervisee feels that she has not been listened to.

Sometimes it might be useful to explain the relevance and say why you bring it up now.

Marjorie tries to diminish the importance of the issue, saying it was only a 'turn of phrase, no offence meant'. Norma: 'Perhaps no offence intended, but it may still be taken. Maybe this is the key to the problem you talked about last time: you know, some patients complaining to the GPs about you. If they pick up that you think they are riff-raff then I do think they have a right to complain.'

Follow up quickly with some support to help the supervisee develop awareness and change, without taking back your challenge or undermining it.
Offer support appropriately.

> Norma senses there is some unacknowledged difficulty underlying the
> prejudice: 'I wonder if you ever feel afraid when you're working in
> the satellite surgery? I know I did when I worked in a similar area'.

There may be times when it is appropriate to drop the subject for a while.
Your aim is to enable the supervisee to develop awareness and to change, not
to win an argument or get your way. Give the supervisee the chance to think
about it and save face, perhaps by changing the subject.

> Marjorie is very red and near to tears but is acting defensively: 'Well,
> of course not, I'm an experienced practice nurse, why should I be
> afraid? And anyway, this isn't what I came here to talk about, this
> is a waste of time.' Norma was aware that Marjorie's aggression may
> reflect the patients' aggression too, but felt this was too much for
> Marjorie to absorb at this time: 'OK, let's put that aside for now. The
> next thing on your agenda was . . .'.

Follow through the challenge if the supervisee is side-tracking or you have
dropped it and the supervisee does not spontaneously return to it herself.

> Marjorie seemed more collected and has been happier discussing
> something less awkward. When that topic seems to have been
> covered, Norma says: 'So does that cover it? Look, I'd like to go
> back to what we were discussing earlier. You know, there's nothing
> wrong in admitting you're afraid sometimes, however experienced
> you are. Perhaps many of the residents of the estate are afraid too,
> especially your vulnerable patients?' They go on to discuss why some
> of Marjorie's patients act aggressively when asked to come to the
> surgery rather than have the district nurse visit. At the next session,
> Marjorie apologises for 'being so bolshy' and seems to have discussed
> her anxieties more openly with her colleagues at the surgery.

Some further examples of challenging

> Blossom, having explored Jacky's concern about the interaction:
> 'I'd just like to go back to what you said about helping the patient
> to turn. You said you didn't bother about using an Immuturn
> frame?' Jacky confirms this. Blossom challenges: 'I think you're
> making a mistake and risking your back. The Trust health and safety
> regulations are very strict about it, there's even EC directives about
> this sort of thing. Have you got a copy of the Trust policy?' Jacky:
> 'Yes, I think so. But we don't often use the Immuturns these days,
> we're all pretty hefty types.' Blossom: 'If this is normal practice on
> your ward I think it's very important that you discuss this with your
> ward manager and get the practice improved as a collective effort.
> How do you think they'd react when you bring it up?' They go on

to discuss how to get cooperation from other nurses and then the doctors.

Pauline to Barbara: 'I can see that the change of approach is difficult for you, but I think that your manager has every right to expect three G grades to cooperate enough to organise their annual leave cover between them. What's the problem between you?' Barbara: 'But I've told you, we tick along very nicely if we keep our distance. We just don't see eye to eye and it's best this way.' Pauline: 'How do you manage to cooperate for other things, like covering clinics if someone's off sick or having to deal with a client crisis?' Barbara: 'Well, the other two box and cox between them, they both have their own large families and are for ever having to take time off for this and that. I'm single, I never have any sick leave and I don't have crises with the families on my caseload, I can anticipate them, I manage my caseload properly. So I keep myself to myself.' Pauline: 'It sounds to me as if there are some difficulties in dealing with differences in ways of managing your caseloads and in your different lifestyles and that leaves you quite isolated.' Barbara: 'You could say that'. Pauline: 'Look, the session's almost over for today, but I'm really concerned for you: I anticipate there may be a crisis looming for you, because your manager would have the right eventually to discipline you if you will not get adequate cover organised for your annual leave and I don't want that to happen to you. Will you think about how you can at least get the roster sorted out soon?' Barbara: 'I suppose so.' Pauline: 'If you'd like an earlier session than the one we've planned for next time, to talk it through, just let me know. I really want to help you prevent this blowing up.' They finish the session and Pauline resolves to take this to her own clinical supervision as she is dreading the next session.

David continues to assert that he has fulfilled his responsibilities in reporting the problem to his manager. Hannah says: 'David, it's really important that you take this further. You really do have a professional ethical responsibility to keep at it, to persist until the abuse has been stopped for good. You are professionally accountable to the UKCC in this instance. Do you understand that?' David: 'Well, what else can I do?' Hannah gives firm advice: 'You should put your concerns in writing to your manager and demand immediate action and, if necessary, send a copy to her manager. I'll help you draft it now if you like.' They go on to work out a letter and Hannah explains that she will have to use the 'exception to confidentiality' groundrule that they agreed at the outset of clinical supervision, in order to check that he has sent it and that some action has been taken.

Zara to Carol: 'Your action plan was that you'd confront Betty about this, but you've been putting it off for months. What's the problem?' Carol talks about the stress involved in plucking up the courage to speak to Betty, anticipating Betty's upset reaction. Zara explains more about why she is pushing the point: 'Well, a lot of your time with me is spent on my supporting you with the stress of dealing with an unnecessarily high workload. I don't think you'll ever be able to manage your time properly until you've confronted Betty and you both have a more equal share of the work. Would it help to look in more detail at what you might say to her?'

Mohammed to Rob: 'You seem to me to be expecting me to instantly come up with a solution to this problem.' Rob: 'Well, that's what you're here for isn't it?' Mohammed: 'I'd like you to think back to the agreement we made in our first session in April. Remember, my role is to help you to think it through and come to your own decision, and yours is to take responsibility for that'. Rob: 'But I've thought it through and I don't know what to do about it.' Mohammed changes to an informative mode and offers to talk him through a problem-solving cycle, making a drawing of the cycle as he speaks. Rob becomes quite interested and the session becomes productive. However, at the beginning of the next session, Rob is a bit late and seems to be back at square one. Mohammed: 'Rob, I get the impression that you are still expecting me to provide instant answers. I wonder if the real problem is that you don't want to be here?' It turns out that Rob feels overwhelmed with the pressure of his work and making the time to get to clinical supervision is a great strain on him and he resents the added pressure. They go on to explore how Rob can manage his time, asking for more help from colleagues and let the manager know about some totally unacceptable and unmanageable aspects of the workload, rather than just struggling on non-assertively.

Pete's challenging question to Danielle (p. 162) led her to realise that she had been especially hard on the agency nurse and eventually she came to the conclusion that she was feeling a bit insecure in her authority as a very young ward manager, because the nurse was much older and more experienced in the field than Danielle was. Had the question not achieved this awareness-raising, Pete might have tried to take it further by asking: 'It sounds to me that you've been especially harsh with this agency nurse and that her confidence goes to pieces when she works with you. What triggers your irritation in particular?'

Fran to Roxanne: 'I haven't heard you speak kindly of any of the parents lately, just criticising. You used to enjoy working with them. I wonder what's gone wrong?' Roxanne blusters for a while then bursts into tears and tells Fran about her recent miscarriage: 'It all seems so unfair, some of these parents talk to their kids as if they didn't really want them, that it's one big nuisance that the child's ill, yet people like me and Nathan are dying to have a child and we're devastated about losing this one. I feel so stupid about getting upset like this, my mum says I'm over-reacting, lots of women have miscarriages.' Fran gives support, pointing out she has a right to be upset and that people often underestimate the impact of a miscarriage. Eventually she brings it back to working with parents. 'So, in spite of feeling so raw about it, how do think you can keep working effectively with parents on the ward? What did you used to enjoy most?' Roxanne talks about showing the parents how to encourage the children to play, in spite of their illness or physical limitations, and what a difference this makes to the child and to the parent–child relationship.

Pitfalls in challenging

Most of the pitfalls arise from the clinical supervisor's own (quite natural) anxiety about challenging: the anxiety can be allowed to get in the way of steering a supportive mid-line between over- or under-doing it.

One of the most common pitfalls seems to be avoidance, putting off making the challenge until it is too late or pussyfooting around, making half-hearted hints, over-using support and catalytic skills and never quite coming to the point. One way to deal with this is to acknowledge your discomfort, such as 'I feel uncomfortable bringing this up, but . . .' or, if you hear yourself waffling, to start off the challenge with 'I'll come to the point . . .'. If the best time for the challenge has passed, you might still retrieve the situation by going back to the point, for example: 'I've been thinking about what you said last time about . . .'.

Sledge-hammering is the opposite: being too harsh, non-supportive and punitive. Sometime this happens because the clinical supervisor has pussy-footed and built up such a level of tension that her belated challenge comes out too strongly. Alternatively, the situation might remind her of something difficult that she herself has experienced. This especially highlights the need for clinical supervisors to have their own supervision. For instance, Pauline realises that her frustration with Barbara is rising and she might go over the top in attacking Barbara's judgement of and resolute isolation from her working-mother colleagues. As a lone parent, she herself had once worked with someone with a similar attitude and found it very difficult. She discusses with her own supervisor how she might be able to remember what she can genuinely support about Barbara without backtracking on her challenge and without becoming one more person that Barbara infuriates and withdraws from.

Inappropriate smiling can result from your nervousness: 'smiling demolition' is when you try to soften a heavy challenge with a smile which contradicts the seriousness of what you are saying. The supervisee can interpret the smile as your enjoying their discomfort. 'Smiling dilution' is when you give a gentle challenge with a smile and the challenge loses its importance, the supervisee cannot take you seriously. Fran knows she has a tendency to smile inappropriately when nervous and she tries to take her facial tension away from her mouth by consciously raising her eyebrows: she cannot easily smile and raise her eyebrows at the same time so this helps.

In an attempt to make the challenge with a light touch, use of humour may end up as a jokey put-down, insensitive tease or sarcastic comment. For example, Pete has a great ability to use a humorous light touch in making even some of the most difficult challenges palatable to his supervisees, but his sense of humour can go too far sometimes. He is aware of how he needs to monitor this to avoid his banter being experienced as mockery. Joking about Danielle being the 'young dragon stalking Ward 10' might be OK when Danielle's worked through the issue of her youth and her authority and not feeling so vulnerable about it, but not until then.

Your anxiety may make you talk too much, saying too much for the supervisee to take in, repeating yourself and not giving the supervisee space to react. If you have a tendency towards this pitfall, it might be helpful to practise giving hypothetical challenges, or to pre-rehearse for a real situation, if you have time. Pauline senses that her anxiety and frustration may lead her to giving Barbara a lecture about the importance of team work in health visiting, so she rehearses some short and to-the-point statements in readiness for the next session with her.

The clinical supervisor's determination to get the issue tackled may lead to a win–lose push, until she has won and the supervisee has lost face. To avoid this pitfall, remember that the purpose of the challenge is to raise awareness and support the supervisee towards change. Developing increased awareness and changing usually take time, so try to give the supervisee space to reflect. If the issue is not urgent, be prepared to drop it temporarily until the supervisee is more ready to work with it. In the situation with Marjorie, Norma would have fallen into this pitfall if she had pushed the point too much while Marjorie was so embarrassed and flustered.

On the other hand, lack of follow-through can make your challenge ineffective. This may happen through timidity, over-sympathising or allowing oneself to be side-tracked by a supervisee who responds to challenge by trying to divert you away from the point. One way to avoid this is to hold the issue in your mind when the discussion moves on, and to come back to it when appropriate. For instance, Fran would have fallen into this pitfall if her support for Roxanne had resulted in her forgetting the ultimate purpose of clinical supervision, i.e. to enhance the quality of practice. Had she not returned to the issue of working effectively with the patient's parents, she would have lacked follow-through.

In this section on the skills and pitfalls of challenging we have focused mainly on some everyday examples and an array of issues that you may need to challenge, in your clinical supervisor role (see Table 6.1). We have deliberately avoided using the most extreme illustrations of the use of challenging to maintain standards and accountability, although nurses often ask if any special considerations apply in clinical supervision. To have included these extremes would have catastrophised the normative principles of clinical supervision rather than balancing it amid the support and growth principles. Dimond (1997a) illustrates the point that dealing with the more extreme cases of discovering dangerous practice is the same as if you had discovered this in any other situation in nursing: you are obliged to put aside any other consideration and ensure the safety of the patient or the public with an

Table 6.1   Pitfalls in challenging in clinical supervision

- AVOIDANCE – Putting off making the challenge until it is too late
- PUSSYFOOTING – Making half-hearted hints, over-using support and catalytic skills and never quite coming to the point
- SLEDGE-HAMMERING – Being too harsh, non-supportive and punitive
- 'SMILING DEMOLITION' – Trying to soften a heavy challenge with a smile which contradicts the seriousness of what you are saying
- 'SMILING DILUTION' – Giving a gentle challenge with a smile and the challenge loses its importance; the supervisee cannot take you seriously
- JOKEY PUT-DOWN – Insensitive tease or sarcastic comment
- TALKING TOO MUCH – Saying too much for the supervisee to take in, repeating yourself and not giving supervisee space to react
- WIN–LOSE PUSH – Inappropriate persistence in order to win and the supervisee loses face
- LACK OF FOLLOW-THROUGH – Inappropriate lack of persistence

appropriate level of urgency. This applies equally to clinical supervision. The clinical supervisor has no more or less responsibility for dealing with inadequate professional standards than any other nurse who discovers such causes for concern.

As a clinical supervisor or member of a clinical supervision group, your use of your skills in giving information, advice and challenge arises from your natural authority as a professional nurse and colleague. The authoritative approach, when linked appropriately with support and catalytic skills, allows for an appropriate symmetry in the clinical supervision relationship that is a fundamental part of the working alliance that we advocated in Chapter 3.

7   *Skills of group clinical supervision*

This chapter looks at the skills required to be a participant in, and to be the facilitator of, a clinical supervision group, but it cannot stand alone: the skills involved in building the working alliance, being a supervisee and clinical supervisor, which we examined in Chapters 3, 4, 5 and 6, are as important in group clinical supervision as they are in one-to-one clinical supervision. As a member of a clinical supervision group, you are building multiple clinical supervision relationships: with each of the other group members, with the facilitator and with the group as a whole. Given that any group develops its own identity, its whole becoming more than just the sum of its parts, you will have a sense of the group as an entity in itself and will also have a relationship with 'the group' which is over and above the relationships you have with individual members. Many of the psychological processes outlined in Chapter 2 also apply to this relationship and can help or hinder its effectiveness, with the added layer of group dynamics to complicate the relationship even further. If the aim of a group is to study these group dynamics, then most of the activity of the group is unstructured, to allow these issues to surface and be enacted. The main purpose of a clinical supervision group is not to study group dynamics; therefore we suggest some structures which aim to help you acknowledge some of the complexity of the group clinical supervision working alliance, and minimise the potential for deeper issues to sabotage the work of the group.

This chapter offers frameworks for understanding and building group skills and some structures for carrying out group clinical supervision that are intended to enable you to work with your clinical supervision group members towards building a secure enough psychological base for effective clinical supervision to take place (see Figure 7.1).

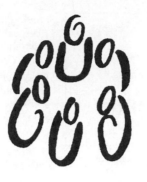

Group members
- supervisee skills
- clinical supervisor skills
- group participation skills

Facilitator
- clinical supervisor skills
- group participation skills
- group facilitation skills

Figure 7.1   Skills needed for effective clinical supervision in a group

Defining group clinical supervision

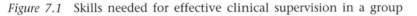

To begin we wish to clarify what group clinical supervision is and what it is not. First, misunderstandings can occur about the concept of a 'group'. We define a 'group' as: three or more people who come together and interrelate cooperatively with each other towards their common purpose. Therefore, a clinical supervision group is: three or more people who come together and interrelate cooperatively with each other towards their common purpose of giving and receiving clinical supervision. (See Figure 7.2.)

For instance, in Room 1 a collection of five people is sitting in a circle receiving information from the speaker about 'Trust guidelines for clinical supervision'. They are not a 'group': although the audience may be sitting in a circle, and they are there for the common purpose of learning about clinical supervision, there is no interaction towards that common purpose: this is a briefing meeting. We are not suggesting there is anything wrong with briefing meetings: combined with written handouts, they are an effective method of passing on information within an organisation, but they are not a clinical supervision group.

In Room 2, a collection of five people is sitting in a circle waiting for their turn to have clinical supervision-type attention from the leader. Again, they are not a *group*: they are in the same place for the same purpose (to get clinical supervision), but are not interrelating specifically towards that goal. They might as well be a queue of people waiting outside the flimsily partitioned office of a clinical supervisor, eavesdropping on what's going on. We cannot see any value in this method: it is a time-consuming way to provide one-to-one clinical supervision.

In contrast, in Room 3, five people are meeting and communicating with each other by taking turns to be the supervisee and using the skills, knowledge, experience and qualities of all those present (including the group facilitator) to provide clinical supervision for each person. This is a clinical supervision *group*.

The second misunderstanding can relate to the nature of the collaborative work a group does together. We have found that some groups which meet

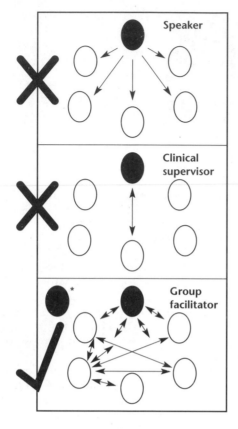

Figure 7.2   Interaction in group clinical supervision

for professional purposes have been mistakenly dubbed clinical supervision, when the work they do together, though valuable, is not actually clinical supervision. For instance, an intensive therapy team which meets to debrief after a traumatic incident on the unit may be doing something essential for the mental health of staff members and for the cohesion of the team, but they are not a clinical supervision group because they are not doing clinical supervision. A group of health visitors who work in isolated rural GP surgeries meet to make human contact, give each other general support, share information about organisational issues and discuss current topics of concern in the profession: they may be having very valid, necessary and constructive meetings, but they are not a clinical supervision group because they are not doing clinical supervision. A group of mental health nurses who are working with a group analyst as facilitator may be getting support and learning a lot about group dynamics, especially about unconscious processes in groups, but they are not a clinical supervision group because they are not doing clinical supervision. A group of staff nurses and students who meet when they are able, during quiet spells in the afternoon, to share their reading of the nursing journals may be functioning very well as a journal group, but they are not a clinical supervision group because they are not doing clinical supervision.

To become clinical supervision groups, these groups would have to have a more regular pattern of planned meetings, fixed months ahead. The membership of the group would need to be fixed in order that there is enough continuity to allow the group members' relationships with each other to develop into a secure enough psychological base. The actual work done together would have to change so that each person gets the chance for in-depth reflection on their own practice and on the part they as individuals play in the complexities and quality of that practice, facilitated in that reflection by the supportive, catalytic, challenging and informative interventions of the other group members.

So, our definition of a clinical supervision group is: three or more people form a fixed membership group and have planned, regular meetings in which each person gets the chance for in-depth reflection on their own practice and on the part they as individuals play in the complexities and quality of that practice, facilitated in that reflection by the other group members.

Skills of group participation

When you are being effective as a group participant, you are using skills of managing your individualistic, competitive and cooperative impulses, and using predominantly collaborative skills in your communication with others in the group.

Individual goals and impulses

It is important to be aware of your own types of individual goals in attending the group and of the impulses which lead you towards those goals. Each type of goal plus its impulse is termed a 'goal structure'. Johnson and Johnson (1987) describe three categories of goal structures: cooperative, individualistic and competitive. They suggest that each person brings all three to any group to which they belong, whether s/he is aware of them or not.

You have a cooperative goal structure when your individual goal is similar to everyone else's in the group, and your goal is not achieved if others do not achieve theirs, e.g. to receive and give effective clinical supervision. Your impulse will therefore be towards ensuring that you have your air time and some useful help from others and that this is reciprocated with everyone in the group.

Your individualistic goal structure is when your individual goal is not related to anyone else's and your achieving yours does not depend on others achieving theirs, e.g. to satisfy your curiosity about what is happening in another unit and find out if the rumours you have heard are true. In this example your impulse would be towards diverting the interaction away from clinical supervision into having a gossip session instead.

Your competitive goal structure is when your individual goal is only achieved if others do not achieve the same, e.g. to be seen as the one who is best at something, such as knowing the most models of clinical supervision, thinking

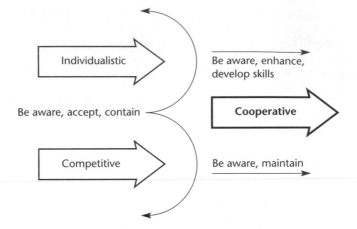

Figure 7.3　Managing your own impulses as a group participant

of solutions to problems or asking the most clever questions. In this example, your impulse would be not so much to help the person having 'air time' for their problem, but to find an opening in which to insert your competitive comment, for maximum effect on your image.

The skills of an effective group participant are those of awareness, acceptance and selective impulse containment and enhancement (see Figure 7.3). Being aware of your own goals and impulses goes hand in hand with self-acceptance: every human being has these impulses and goals and you are not a bad person if you become aware of your negative ones. You can use your awareness to enhance and give full rein to your cooperative goals and impulses for your own and the group's benefit, while containing your individualistic and competitive ones. A group participant who is unable to contain their individualistic and competitive urges will damage the group and render it ineffective. Next we will look at how you can enhance and maintain your cooperative impulses as a group participant.

Skills of cooperation

To set the context of the group participation skills that we suggest are important for cooperation in a group, we need to consider the dynamics of an effective clinical supervision group. There are many phase theories which describe the energy phases of groups. Jacques (1991) provides a good overview of a wide range of them (but beware of playing competitive 'let's see who knows the most group dynamics theories' games!). Our clinical supervision version simplifies the main phases referred to by most of the theorists (see Figure 7.4). We find there are three main enabling phases which support the collaborative clinical supervision work of an effective clinical supervision group: first, settling, then energising, then, after the collaborative clinical supervision work, completing (see Figure 7.4).

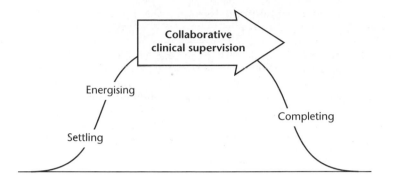

Figure 7.4 The enabling phases of an effective clinical supervision group

If these enabling phases are effectively attended to by the group, then the quality of the collaboration and the work of the group towards its purpose is greatly enhanced. Collaboration goes wrong when the enabling phases are not attended to.

There are also many role theories which describe the various roles that group members can take in a group. Belbin's (1981) is probably the most widely quoted, though it is most useful when applied to work teams of eight to ten people. Randall and Southgate (1980) incorporate role theory into their phase theory. They suggest that individual group members are each likely to have a tendency to contribute more at one or other of the phases of group energy. We adapt their framework here. As a clinical supervision group participant, it can be useful to clarify your own tendency and to take this into account when working in your group: that is, do you have more skills in 'settling', 'energising' or 'completing'?

People who are predominantly skilled at settling tend to be good at the skills of establishing and maintaining relationships. They are the people who make sure that people get welcomed and introduced and help people feel included in what's going on: they chat easily and the group relaxes. Settling skills include checking that everyone understands the purpose of the group, establishing and maintaining groundrules (such as those in Table 7.1). They also include clarifying what resources are needed and available for doing the work together, offering relevant new information needed for the collaborative work and ensuring everyone understands it. Suggesting a plan or 'order of play' as a framework for the group's activity and providing 'tools' to help people grasp what is going on are both settling skills. People skilled at settling are able to influence other group members through sharing useful information and through their openness. They are easy to get to know in a group, being comfortable with the skills of self-disclosure and of listening to others non-judgementally.

If the 'settlers' in a group are in a majority, or are especially influential and the settling phase goes on too long, then the group atmosphere becomes too comfortable. It can degenerate into non-productive, cosy chat and eventually

Table 7.1 Examples of additional groundrules for group clinical supervision

---

1 *Confidentiality*: the groundrule outlined in Chapter 4 is augmented by the clause that anything personal which anyone shares is kept confidential to the context in which it was disclosed, i.e. any work in pairs or subgroups is kept to that context and not disclosed in the whole group, unless permission is given to pass it on. There are two exceptions: disclosure of unsafe or illegal practice

2 *Autonomy and choice*: each person can decide for themselves how much to disclose or keep private and can stop any process that is causing undue pressure on them

3 *Speaking for self*: trying to speak in the first person, i.e. 'I think/feel/find in my experience . . .' rather than 'you', 'one' or 'we' when speaking about own opinions, feelings and experiences

4 *No put-downs*: no judgements about other colleagues' personalities, feelings, shared experiences, vulnerabilities

5 *Commitment*: making the group clinical supervision sessions a priority and bending over backwards to make the necessary arrangements to attend punctually each time, sending a message if unable to do so. Also, being willing to take what is, for you, some risk in speaking up in the group, and being prepared to feel somewhat awkward at times in order to try something different and so to learn

6 *Reciprocity*: each person taking part agrees to take their turn to be both giver and recipient of clinical supervision

---

the group energy falls flat. People feel smothered, there is avoidance of nitty-gritty discussion and a fear of rocking the boat through disagreement or surfacing conflict. There is little motivation to get the work done so the group action is half-hearted, if done at all.

If you are skilled at settling, your initiatives are very much needed in the establishment of the group, when people do not know each other well and are especially nervous. Your taking a lead near the beginning of each group session will be useful, to help everyone put aside the busy-ness of activities before the session and settle into being a group again. During the other phases of the group, your contributions can continue to remind the group of its purpose and groundrules, and your ability for self-disclosure and listening can oil the wheels of real communication. Look out for any tendency to 'mother hen' the group: if you are encouraging the group to linger over or slide back into a cosy settling phase, then sit back and let the 'energisers' take more of a lead, however uncomfortable this might make you feel.

Skilled energisers are likely to feel impatient with the settling phase and want to get on with things. They do not like sitting around gently chatting and want to charge the group with energy. Energising skills include being able to excite a meeting with enthusiasm and being full of ideas and creative possibilities. They also include being able to stimulate some creative tension through playing 'devil's advocate', stirring up some indignation in the less energetic until they take a more active part. Making logical and intuitive connections and formulating and articulating arguments are energising skills, along with the quality of being not easy to put down. Skilled energisers are able to influence other group members through reasoned argument, persuasion and impassioned speeches. They can usually assert their own needs, for example, for 'air time' and can be good advocates for others in the group who are less assertive.

If people predominantly skilled at energising dominate the proceedings, the more reflective people give up when they can't get a word in edgeways or when their constructive contributions are undermined or shouted down by compulsive 'devil's advocates'. There can be too much non-focused discussion, with ideas going in too many different directions, with some group members becoming overwhelmed by it all. The quality of listening falls and some people get locked in endless argument whilst those who attempt to break the cycle get attacked for their efforts. A cold atmosphere develops and there's a reluctance to attend next time. Again, the task of the group does not get done with full cooperation and is therefore not done properly, if at all.

If you are skilled at energising, your input is very much needed in the energising phase of the group, but try not to jump in too near the beginning or get too carried away during the energising phase. Attempt to focus your and the group's energy onto the task of effective clinical supervision; or, if you find it hard to get focused, allow others to do this. Your contribution in any of the other phases can be helpful to keep the energy going or move along a group that becomes stuck. The combination of skilled settlers and energisers taking leadership roles in the group can make for a very positive and energetic start to a group, and the collaboration in doing clinical supervision together can develop very well from this basis. However, when the main body of the work has been done, the completers can help tie it all together.

Completers are usually calm and reflective and possibly the quietest people in the first few phases of the group. They are the people who can see the totality of the work that has gone on and their group participation skills include clarifying themes, making summaries, clarifying decisions that have been made, drawing conclusions and making final links. Their 'helicopter' vision may lead them to see more clearly the process of the group and this can be useful feedback to the others. They help to cool out a meeting and help clarify what has and has not been achieved. They may be able to suggest plans that need to be made for next time and a way of ending the meeting on a positive note.

In contrast with the other two enabling phases, we find that it is common in groups of nurses for the completing phase to be under- rather than over-emphasised. This leads to puzzlement for some group members about what was achieved, or feelings of being taken for granted. The energy is focused into rushing off to the next thing without finishing the group and there is difficulty arranging further meetings while half the group are rushing out of the door. There is little regard for group successes and the group can become undervalued, with decreasing motivation to attend each time. In contrast, in academic nursing settings, there are often more completers in a group and the pitfall can be 'analysis-paralysis' whereby analysis of the group's work and process is drawn out beyond its usefulness.

We find when working with practitioners that completers often undervalue and hold back their contribution. If you are predominantly skilled at completing, it is important that you push yourself forward at the appropriate time as your perspective can stimulate and clarify an essential part of the learning that is done in the clinical supervision group. During other phases, you can contribute positively by sharing your 'helicopter' vision of the proceedings, validating the way the group is working together or highlighting when it is going off track.

This framework for looking at roles in a group is not fixed: we do not anticipate that you will always use your collaborative skills in the same way every time your clinical supervision group meets. As you consider the three enabling phases and the roles that people play in a group, you are likely to find that you are able to contribute to more than one phase. You might find that your style of participation differs according to the people you are with or according to how you are feeling on a certain day. We suggest this framework as a way of raising your awareness of the skills you already have, the possible pitfalls in terms of your effect on the group's energy and flagging up some group participation skills that you may wish consciously to develop in order that your clinical supervision group can have an effective balance between the three enabling phases of group energy.

Skills of group facilitation

The person whose role is to facilitate a clinical supervision group needs to have more than the clinical supervision skills we outlined in Chapters 4, 5 and 6: group facilitator skills are also necessary in order to ensure that the group is effective. Our definition of a group facilitator is: someone who works with a group to enable the members to communicate and cooperate with each other towards achieving their common purpose. Bentley's (1994: 31) definition emphasises the autonomy of the group: '[Group] Facilitation is the provision of opportunities, resources, encouragement and support for the group to succeed in achieving its objectives and to do this through enabling the group to take control and responsibility in the way they proceed'. Heron's (1989: 11) definition highlights the appointment and voluntary acceptance of the group facilitator and focuses on groups where their common purpose is to learn from their experience together:

> A group facilitator is a person who has the role of helping participants to learn in an experiential group. The facilitator will normally be formally appointed to this role by whatever organisation is sponsoring the group. And the group members will voluntarily accept the facilitator in this role. By experiential group I mean one in which learning takes place through an active and aware involvement of the whole person – as a spiritual thinking, feeling, choosing, energetically and physically embodied being.

These concepts of 'group facilitator' underpin the framework we are presenting here.

Some clinical supervision groups have a regular facilitator whose role is to facilitate the group each time and does not take their turn to receive clinical supervision: they have theirs elsewhere. The options for who should be this person are similar to those we have outlined in Chapter 8, with the added

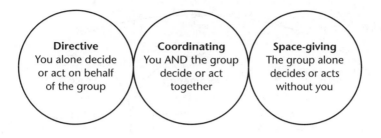

Figure 7.5   Three modes of group facilitation

requirement that they should have skills in group facilitation. We emphasise that this person should not have any line management relationship with anyone in the group: our rationale for this is given in Part I. In other groups, members take turns to be the group facilitator. There are advantages and disadvantages in having an outside group facilitator or being peer-facilitated and these are outlined in Chapter 8.

As a framework for examining the skills of a group facilitator, we offer an adaptation of Heron's (1989) styles of group facilitation (see Figure 7.5). It focuses on the question: who manages the tasks and the process of the group? In a clinical supervision group, attention needs to be paid not only to the clinical supervision that is given and received but also how the process of communication and cooperation between group members is handled. It suggests three main options you have as facilitator at any point when deciding what needs to be done:

1 to be directive and take charge of some of the tasks or process on your own, *for and on behalf of the group*
2 to be coordinating and manage some of the tasks or process *with the group*
3 to be space-giving and let the group manage the tasks or process *for themselves.*

The three modes are not static: you can move flexibly from mode to mode as appropriate, from moment to moment. Examples of this flow are given later in the chapter. Overall, a rule of thumb in clinical supervision groups is to move from short periods of being directive, in order to set the scene; to being predominantly coordinating; then predominantly space-giving when group members become settled and able to communicate and cooperate effectively with little active intervention from you as group facilitator.

There is no intention to suggest that any one of the three is 'better' than another: all have their time and place. Some nurses practising group facilitator skills can sometimes feel uncomfortable with coordinating or space-giving since they believe that they are not 'doing' enough in these modes. Others can feel uncomfortable with the directive mode since they believe that group facilitators should be totally non-directive, that a group should wallow in chaos until it finds its own level. Our view is that these positions are too extreme. The urge towards too much direction is a common but mistaken tendency in a hierarchical culture such as nursing, and destroys the effectiveness

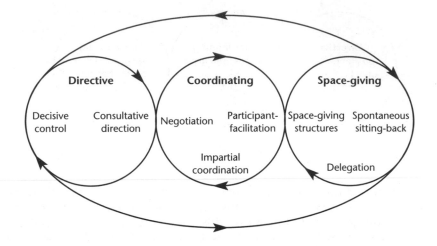

Figure 7.6 Flowing between the three modes of group facilitation

of a clinical supervision group: motivation to participate and turn up to sessions diminishes. This tendency is a two-way process if the group facilitator is in a position of managerial authority over the group members: however non-directive the facilitator tries to be at the outset, the group members will tend to respond better to the more directive interventions and subliminally push the facilitator into being directive.

On the other hand, there is an urge towards extreme non-direction in facilitators of some clinical supervision groups. This sometimes seems to arise from the 1970s backlash against hierarchical control in which the pendulum swung too far the other way. It can also arise from misapplication of some group analytic methods which are intended for group therapy, not learning groups such as clinical supervision. Again, too much non-direction can make a clinical supervision group ineffective and people lose their motivation to participate and attend.

Looking at these modes, we urge you to develop skills which allow for a flow between being directive and being non-directive from moment to moment when facilitating a clinical supervision group (see Figure 7.6). We focus on the directive mode first.

Directive group facilitation

The group facilitator directs, does things and makes decisions for and on behalf of the group. You take responsibility for and make decisions about some of the tasks or the process. However, these decisions and actions are done with the intention that they will ultimately enable the group to cooperate more in working together and therefore need less direction from you. So, for instance, while you may be directive in giving some necessary information, you keep it brief and you're careful not to project so much charismatic energy that the group members become captivated into becoming an attentive audience.

This mode can be sub-divided into two: decisive control is the most direct-ive, and consultative direction slightly less so. Decisive control is where you make the decision or carry out some action without any consultation of the group beforehand, perhaps spelling out take-it-or-leave-it options, maintain-ing your bottom line, insisting on something which you know to be import-ant. This is all done in a way which gives people the genuine choice to accept it or not.

> Lisa decides the venue of the first clinical supervision group meeting. It would be a waste of time for her to send memos to the group participants to coordinate their views on a venue: someone needs to get on with it or the group will never get started.

> In a more established group, Bryony is facilitating a group clinical supervision session in which Karen is being disruptive: she is bad-tempered and is being negative about everything, including being destructively critical of one member of the group who is feeling vulnerable. Bryony has tried a supportive approach, giving Karen the chance to talk about what's making her so grumpy, but to no avail. So Bryony decides to confront her: 'Karen, it seems to me that your grumpiness and negativity are getting in the way of what this group is here to do. I'd like you to work more cooperatively, or at least stop hindering others in doing so, or accept some support for what's bugging you.' Karen sulks for a while, but at least the others are able to get on with the work. She later apologises and during the following meeting is able to accept some support for the very considerable stress she is under in her job.

Consultative direction is when you collect and listen to information and views from group members and make your decision afterwards, whether or not you adapt your decision according to the information you've received.

> Lisa invites potential group members to let her know which dates they would be available for the first few in the series of clinical supervision sessions. She decides the best dates which suit the most people, including herself.

> In the last few minutes of Bryony's group clinical supervision session, there is little time left to plan the next meeting (this group likes to have an 'order of play' worked out beforehand). She asks which group members wish to have 'air time' and what their preferences are for the order in which they work. She bears in mind what they have said and then decides the sequence.

The pitfalls involved in being directive are to do with being directive too much or too little or in an inappropriate manner. Too much of this mode can result in a passive and dependent group (though sometimes they may be content with this, since it may be what they are used to) or a resentful/sabotaging group. Group members lose their self-direction and potential for cooperating together. Taking on an 'expert' role in group clinical supervi-sion, perhaps by making a lot of clinical supervisor interventions, can leave the group expecting that you are there to do the job rather than to enable the group to do it for themselves: it can become a 'taking turns to have one-to-one clinical supervision, in front of an audience' format instead of true group clinical supervision.

Too much skilled direction of the group process can turn the group into amazed observers, marvelling at your skill and going along with you, but feeling that they could never do what they are doing unless you are directing them.

Your manner may slip into an authoritarian, aggressive, abusive, bossy, critical or patronising style. Most of us have had plenty of such role models in nursing. On the other hand, you may develop a charismatic, captivating style and people are happy to follow you, or at least, are unwilling to challenge your directiveness because they like you. This can be equally disabling of real communication within a group.

At the other end of the scale, your manner may be apologetic about being directive. This flabbiness can leave the group feeling sorry for you and going along with you to make you feel better, or irritated by your ineffectualness and likely to sabotage. It is necessary to be directive at times, and some facilitators feel they are failing when they are doing so, perhaps because of a legacy from the days when facilitator training veered too much towards the non-directive. Too little direction can create unnecessary confusion and lack of safety, and deprive the group of some of your knowledge and expertise or support and protection.

Coordinating mode of group facilitation

Here the facilitator shares power, does things and decides with the group. You guide and enable collaborative action and decision making. There are three main types of coordinating, in decreasing order of directiveness: negotiation, impartial coordination, participant-facilitation.

You can negotiate with the group, share your own views which may be influential but not final, and enable group members to negotiate with you and with each other.

> Lisa suggests a 'learning set' structure for the clinical supervision sessions and receives comments. Two group members want to push the design away from clinical supervision towards an unstructured support group. Lisa spells out her bottom line, which is the need to have some pre-agreed structure, such as set amounts of air time for each person agreed beforehand, but she is willing to negotiate on other aspects, such as making the support element of the feedback explicit. Together she and the group adapt the structure to take in her concerns and those of the two group members.

> Bryony's group has degenerated from giving air time to one group member, Sam, into a general discussion in which no one is listening to one another, especially not to Sam. Bryony says, 'I get the impression that you're discussing red herrings and having difficulties listening to each other. Why do you think that's happening?' The

group discusses this and eventually agrees that the subjects they are discussing are interesting but are diversions from Sam's problem and that their listening has gone down the plughole. Bryony goes on: 'I wonder if it's because the problem that Sam brought has shocked you and reminded you of your own limitations but that's too painful to admit? That's my interpretation of the situation: what's yours?' Bryony and the group discuss this and, in effect, negotiate a common understanding of the group process.

Impartial coordination is when you actively facilitate the group's inter-action towards their objective, but you do not have any direct input your-self into the topic/task they are working on. This is often the official role of a chairperson at a meeting (though in practice the chairperson often loses impartiality and tries to influence the outcome). It is especially useful when facilitating in this mode to pay attention to the three enabling phases of group energy that were outlined earlier in the chapter and draw in or inter-rupt group members who have strong tendencies to a particular type of energy, according to the phase of the meeting.

Some members of Lisa's group wish to finish the clinical supervision meeting early, so the whole group starts arguing about this. Lisa has nothing to say about the actual decision since they are progressing well through the plan for the session. She intervenes only occasionally to ensure that the quieter people have the chance to have their say. Then she points out to them that they seem to have come to a decision yet the discussion is going round in circles unnecessarily.

Bryony's group has become stuck in gloom about Sam's problem. She asks Jean (who is usually full of ideas) an open question to refocus attention on the problem-solving cycle and actively encourages the other members to add their thoughts. She does not offer any answers to the questions.

Participant-facilitation is when you take an active part in the process, sharing your own contribution as if you were a participant, not actively facilitating but modelling good participation.

Lisa's clinical supervision group is working in two groups of three at either end of the room. Lisa joins in as a participant in one of the sub-groups. However, she has her antennae out, having some awareness for how well the other triad is coping and she is ready to change mode if necessary.

At the beginning of the first meeting after the Christmas break, Bryony suggests people take a turn at saying their hopes and dreads about the clinical supervision sessions in the coming year. She takes a turn as a participant in this exercise by sharing hers.

Again, the pitfalls in coordinating are about using this mode too much, too little or in an inappropriate manner. Too much can waste time and effort when some direction is appropriate. You may be avoiding being directive (especially when challenge is needed) because you want to be liked. Not moving on to space-giving can result in what Heron (1989) describes as 'a subtle kind of nurturing control which inhibits true self-direction'. Your always being part of the process in such a likeable way can stop them doing it on their own when they are capable. Too much skilled coordination can again leave the group amazed at your skill and dependent on you to coordinate their activities rather than move towards autonomy.

You might slip into a manipulative approach, 'facipulation', giving the appearance of enabling the group, but actually getting them to decide/think/act exactly as you want, without laying your cards on the table. A common example is when the facilitator is writing things up on a flip chart, ostensibly to collect the group's ideas but actually only writing up the points s/he had in mind. This causes cynicism and reduces commitment to participate.

Too little coordination can mean that the group is being directed too much or feels abandoned to get on with it, or swings between those two extremes, without the intermediate stage of establishing how to work together cooperatively with your support.

Space-giving mode of group facilitation

Here the facilitator gives the group the freedom to find their own way, do the work of the group themselves, sort out their own difficulties, make their own mistakes and learn from them. Space is given for group-directed decision making and action. This is not intended to be a laissez-faire option: you choose the time when they are ready and do not abandon the group to get on with it, but instead let them know where and when you will be available to them if they need you or want to draw you in. You have three main options in aiming to be space-giving: setting up space-giving structures, delegating some for the facilitation and spontaneous sitting back.

Space-giving structures give the group members the chance to work in pairs, small groups or in the whole group without your presence, but you need to be clear about where you will be so that you can be available in the room or nearby should they wish to consult you.

> Lisa is using a 'hands off' approach to the clinical supervision in her group. She has set up pairs, where the group members have a period of one and a half hours. After checking that they understand the task, she leaves them in privacy to take turns to have 45 minutes air time with the other taking the clinical supervisor role. She clarifies where she will be and that she will be available if they want some help.

> Bryony's energetic clinical supervision group are having some more problems: two group members, Pat and Eva, seem to have some unfinished conflicts to resolve and are taking up the group's time with irrelevant bickering. She suggests that they have half an hour to sort it out in privacy whilst the group gets on with its work, and report back to the group afterwards. Again, she is not involved in

their interaction but she states where and when she will be available to help if necessary.

Delegation is a second option for space-giving. This is when you delegate some aspect of the facilitator's role to a specific person or persons in the group.

Lisa identifies a time-keeper in each pair for the co-supervision structure and asks them to ensure that the pair have equal air time each and that they reconvene at the agreed time for the last part of the group session.

Bryony's group has been discussing the issue of very differing interruption rates between the men and women. It is agreed that one group member will monitor the subsequent rates of contributions and interruptions for a set period, and report periodically, especially if there is a recurrence of the problem they had originally.

A third option for space-giving is when you spontaneously sit back when the group are doing fine without your intervention, or are quite capable of working through any issues that arise out of your lack of intervention. You maintain your concentration on the group process but you give your support through silent attention.

Lisa has been coordinating the sharing of what they have learned from their clinical supervision session that day. She says nothing for over five minutes, because they are doing well at cooperating with each other in their sharing and discussion.

Bryony has been discussing with the group some of the problems they have been having in keeping to the point and in doing effective clinical supervision together. She stays in the circle but is silent while they consider what they have learned in previous discussions they have had with her about their group process and how they can prevent these blocks in their next session. They get tense but she gives supportive space for them to work through it themselves. They come up with an excellent plan for the next session, that they own and to which they seem to be very committed.

The pitfalls of space-giving in group facilitation can again be described as either too much or too little of this approach or using an inappropriate manner. Too much space-giving may degenerate into a laissez-faire approach, abandoning the group without adequate preparation, facilities or backup support. This is likely to result in the group wallowing in confusion, misconception, ignorance, defensiveness, avoidance of the task, chaos, abuse, negative hierarchies or leadership battles. Too little space-giving stifles the group's potential. They become dependent on the facilitator to guide or rescue them from the inevitable difficulties of working collectively, and the potential creativity of a cooperative clinical supervision group is not sufficiently explored. Their sense of ownership and commitment to the task can diminish. The manner of your space-giving could be punitive. Your underlying message could be, for instance, 'So you think you know it all, then get on with it without me and see what a mess you make'; or 'If you can't be bothered then I can't either'.

Putting it all together

You will move between the three modes of group facilitation from moment to moment as you work with the clinical supervision group. Most of the time you will not be aware of your intentions or the skills you are using to facilitate. However, this three-mode framework can help you to focus your thoughts when planning and when things are not going too well.

> During the first meeting of the clinical supervision group, Lisa identifies the areas which she considers need to be covered during the first meeting, including sharing hopes and fears, previous experiences of clinical supervision, aims of their meetings, groundrules, practicalities such as timing. She takes about five minutes to outline these and list them on a flip chart as a starting point for the agenda. (Decisive control: she's deciding they need to draw up an agenda.)
>
> She then throws it open for discussion and asks the group some open questions to encourage them to react to her proposed agenda. She gets no response and the long silence is uncomfortable. She rephrases the question and still there is no response. (Attempting negotiation: she was aiming to get a joint agenda.)
>
> She realises that the group members are not yet ready to speak out in the whole group and suggests they talk in pairs about 'What I want from this clinical supervision group' and 'What we need to sort out as a group so I can get what I want', discussing these trigger points together in privacy. (Space-giving structure.)
>
> Bringing them back together, she collects points from each pair, noticing which points had an impact, from the non-verbal reactions of the other group members. She invites specific people who reacted non-verbally to say something: 'You looked interested in what Frank had to say, Barbara. What's your view?' Then she signalled with her hand for Barbara to speak directly to Frank, rather than to herself. (Impartial coordination.)
>
> The discussion gets underway and she sits quietly enjoying the way the group are sharing their ideas, experiences and feelings. They go off the point a little but it seems important to let them get to know each other. (Spontaneous space-giving.)
>
> After a while, she summarises their discussion, adds two points to the list of topics to be covered and starts a list of groundrules, writing in two that arose spontaneously during the discussion. (Negotiation.)
>
> She focuses on establishing groundrules: 'Groundrules seem the most important topic for you at this point, so let's look at them in more detail (consultative direction). What other groundrules would you like to have?' She encourages people to contribute and writes up

what they say. She adds one groundrule that she would like to have, then asks people to clarify a little more what they meant by each point, checks if everyone understands and then if everyone agrees to the list of groundrules as their contract for working together as a clinical supervision group (negotiation.)

Lisa then suggests they focus on sharing experiences of clinical supervision (consultative direction) and invites each person in turn to let the others know what their previous experiences of clinical supervision have been. She takes her turn (participant-facilitation). And so on.

Bryony is facilitating the next clinical supervision group session. Last time, they decided to have one person 'presenting' an issue and having 45 minutes of the group's time to reflect in depth. Bryony stays silent while Karen, a senior sister on a cardiac surgery ward, recounts a traumatic experience (spontaneous sitting back). Karen describes how the family of a seriously ill patient try to abduct the patient against his will to take him back to their home country to die, becoming verbally abusive and threatening towards Karen and the registrar when they intervene. Hospital security staff and eventually the police were involved. Having heard the account, the group are stunned and silent. A few tentative attempts at support are made but these come out in the form of factual questions and do not seem to be experienced as supportive by Karen; in fact, she reacts rather defensively as if the questions imply that she has not dealt with all aspects of the situation.

Bryony manages to step back from the situation and asks the group, 'Having heard Karen's account of this very difficult situation, what strengths did you notice she used in dealing with it?' She then encourages group members to direct their explicitly supportive comments directly to Karen: rather than saying '*She* did well with . . .' to say '*You* did well with . . .' (impartial facilitation). This results in more explicit support and Bryony says nothing as they are doing well (spontaneous sitting back). Later, the group members seem to be using questions focused on problem solving inappropriately, since all action had been taken and plans for the future were fully in place. Bryony realises that it was more appropriate to focus on helping Karen to reflect on her learning from the experience: she suggests this and asks the group to bear in mind a 'learning from experience' cycle that they had used previously (consultative direction). She then uses the framework as a way of focusing a question to Karen to help her reflect, and to help the group members to understand what she is getting at (participant-facilitation).

Others in the group then take over helping Karen through the most appropriate stages of reflecting on the experience and on what she and her staff could learn from the perspective of a few weeks' hindsight. This goes well so Bryony sits back and says nothing (spontaneous sitting back). And so on.

Some structures which might be used or adapted in clinical supervision groups

Learning sets

A learning set is made up of four to six people and a group facilitator who meet at least monthly for at least three months to explore the complex workplace problems or learning issues of each group member in turn, each meeting taking up one whole day. The set membership can be homogeneous or varied: all at a similar level in the same organisation; all at a similar level in different organisations; a vertical slice through some levels of the same organisation; a combination of people from client and provider groups; unidisciplinary partners in the provision of a service; multidisciplinary partners in the provision of a service; any group who feel they can work together in this way.

Background of learning sets

Revans (1982) worked as a management consultant with the newly nationalised Coal Board, just after the Second World War. Engineers and miners were frustrated with expert-led change management and Revans set up action learning sets with mining engineers to increase the practical relevance of change processes, with considerable success. Although Revans found difficulty in gaining acceptance of the action learning approach in organisations and in higher education until the late 1960s, learning sets are now widely accepted as a valuable approach to management and organisational development.

Meanwhile, humanistic psychology emerged as a 'third force' in psychology in the 1950s and 1960s (behaviourism and psychoanalysis being the first two). Humanistic psychology emphasises the individual, subjective interpretation of experience and saw people as free decision makers who could learn and change according to their own wishes. It has a particular emphasis on affective learning, i.e. learning about becoming aware of and constructively handling emotions rather than repressing them under an over-emphasis on intellect. 'Self managed learning sets' developed out of the humanistic psychology movement. It borrowed the structures of learning sets pioneered by Revans to give a framework for a humanistic approach to learning, to be applied in educational as well as occupational settings.

Learning sets are not useful when:

- specific knowledge or skills are best taught by an expert
- people attending are not motivated to learn, not willing to disclose their vulnerabilities, believing that they have no more to learn, etc.
- set members are dependent on having a 'chalk and talk' teacher rather than a facilitator and cannot adapt to this style of learning from peers.

Typical format of a learning set meeting

This relates to the enabling phases we identified earlier in this chapter.

Phase 1 (Settling and Energising): each person speaks in turn, taking a few minutes to share current top-of-the-head preoccupations, news, progress with any action plans made at the last meeting. Support and challenge are given to individuals about how they followed through their action plans. This phase might take about half an hour.

Phase 2 (Collaborative work): each person in turn has the same length of time to have the attention and help of the other members. The person in the 'hot seat' defines how they can most use the time fruitfully and the rest comply as long as it is within their capabilities, ethics, any common agreement about content or process, etc. Each person has at least an hour for in-depth reflection, and there is a lunch break.

Phase 3 (Completing): about half an hour is spent on debriefing, reflecting on the process of the meeting, acknowledging achievements and learning, tying up ends, planning next meetings and ending.

The group facilitator is an outsider to the set and is experienced in group facilitation, though not usually with specific technical or clinical expertise in the area of work done by set members. She is a facilitator of the process and has no direct input into the problems which set members present to the group. She may give guidance on factors affecting the process of communicating and collaborating in the set. For instance, she might provide relevant theoretical underpinning of the process, structures for working together, guidance on how to be appropriately helpful to each 'hot seat' person and ways of understanding and dealing with process blocks and difficulties.

The content of the work done by the learning set
The opportunity that a learning set provides is best utilised when the content of what is brought to the group by individual members includes most of these features:

- it is directly part of the individual's life ('I am part of this issue/problem and it is part of me')
- it is too big for tidy solutions
- it involves 'problems' (i.e. with no single 'best' solution) rather than 'puzzles' (i.e. with one 'best' solution that can be gleaned from an expert)
- it involves multiple factors and human relationships
- it is a real-life issue which needs to be dealt with now.

The type of topics that an individual can bring can be agreed at the outset as: totally up to each person on each occasion the set meets, or part of a joint work project or personal learning theme. For instance, members of an action learning set which is concerned with a change management programme in an organisation will bring examples of complex problems related to that change programme. A self-managed learning set which is made up of people on a professional training course might agree to bring examples of problems in applying the course theory to professional practice.

Sponsors are an essential part of the learning set structure. If the learning set is made up of people from within the same organisation, they may have one sponsor from within the management structure of that organisation. If members are from different work settings, then each set member has a person in their own organisation or from their client group. The sponsor helps to identify problems to be explored in the learning set and has an investment in gaining a solution and provides backup and support in the workplace. They may help provide work-based motivation to put action plans into practice and may be able to open doors to the resources necessary to do this.

Guidelines for using the learning set format as part of a group clinical supervision session

Establish in advance the roles to be taken, i.e. who will be the 'air time' person, other learning set members and the group facilitator. You might want to have an observer to identify the skills being used and the pitfalls. Allocate at least one hour to the learning set process, divided into: seven minutes settling/energising time, at least 45 minutes for the 'air time' person to share an issue and for the other group members to collaborate in providing clinical supervision, and then eight minutes for the completing phase. If you have an observer, you will need to allocate additional time for feedback, perhaps ten minutes.

'Air time' person: your task includes planning in advance to bring a complex topic which relates to you in real life upon which you'd like to reflect with the help of these learning set members. Guidelines for choosing topics are given in Chapter 4. Explain it as clearly as you can, perhaps mapping it out on a flip chart so that the group members can easily follow. Allow the group members to help you reflect in depth on the issue. If you find that you are getting overwhelmed by the number of questions or amount of advice, then say so and ask them to give you more space.

Learning set members: your task includes taking part in the 'settling/ energising' phase by, for instance, checking that everyone knows what to do, finding out what each person wants to get out of the session, sharing news since meeting last, sharing progress on action plans made last time and so on. In the collaborative clinical supervision phase, give the 'air time' person space to outline the issue in their own words before you begin questioning. You can take notes if this helps you. Listen and show you are listening non-verbally and make explicit statements of support before you ask any questions or challenge. Use support, catalytic and challenging skills to enable the 'air time' person to explore the issue in depth. Refrain from giving any advice or information until later on in the session AND ONLY IF IT IS WANTED (check if you are not sure). Ensure that you do not swamp the 'air time' person by competing with other learning set members to support, question, give advice, information, challenge, etc. Take part in the completing phase by sharing what was highlighted for you personally from this experience of working like this and any suggestions you have for using or adapting this structure in the future.

Group facilitator: your task is to guide the group through the settling/ energising, collaborative clinical supervision and completing phases, trying to keep to the times suggested. Ensure that the 'air time' person is given space and explicit support to outline the issue before people start questioning and that they are not swamped with too much questioning, advice, information, challenge, etc. Interrupt when this is beginning to happen. Ensure that the group work stays focused on the issue the 'air time' person brings, not turning the exercise into a general discussion on the topic. If this begins to happen, interrupt and remind them that each person will have a chance to have a say about their own personal involvement in the topic during the winding down phase. Notice the interactions in the group, sit back if all is going well, or take part as a clinical supervisor if appropriate. If the group and the 'air time' person seem stuck, raise this as a problem and suggest a way of dealing with it or encourage the group to think of a way to deal with being stuck.

Observer: your task is to sit back from the group and observe the supervisee skills that the person in the hot seat is using, the clinical supervisor and group participant skills the learning set members are using and the group facilitator's skills. Identify any pitfalls and give feedback at the end.

Self and peer review

Self and peer review is a reciprocal process, carried out in pairs or groups, by which you:

- agree upon one aspect of professional life which you have in common
- generate the criteria for effectiveness in carrying out this aspect of professional life
- take turns to share your own self-assessment and receive supportive and constructively critical feedback from your colleague(s)
- make an action plan for development in this aspect of professional life.

Self and peer review was first described by Heron (1972) and has since been used in a variety of settings. Boud and Kilty (1983) provide guidelines for its use among teachers and researchers working in higher education. Heron (1981) describes its use with NHS Regional Education and Training Officers (educators of doctors) doing clinical audits. It is a model recommended by Pedler *et al.* (1991) for companies taking on the 'Learning Company' principles. The Institute for the Development of Human Potential pioneered its use as the assessment and accreditation method in their training of group facilitators, and various counselling training institutes have since adopted it. In nurse education, we have used it as a valuable adjunct to tutor assessments of students and staff appraisal schemes. We have also used it as a needs assessment and motivating tool for experienced staff embarking (initially unwillingly) upon a staff development programme. We have also used it as a team building tool, for bringing concerns about each other's work out into the open in a constructive and supportive way (Figure 7.7).

Self-assessment is the fundamental element of the self and peer review process, indeed a most important component of a professional person's development: without commitment to your own learning and development, any educational or management process imposed from outside cannot work. Clinical supervision which does not have this at its core is likely to have but transitory effects.

Gregory (1989: 2) states the aims of self-assessment:

The aim of self assessment is to enable the person to integrate the ideal self (i.e. the fantasy of what I could be/would like to be, which tends to

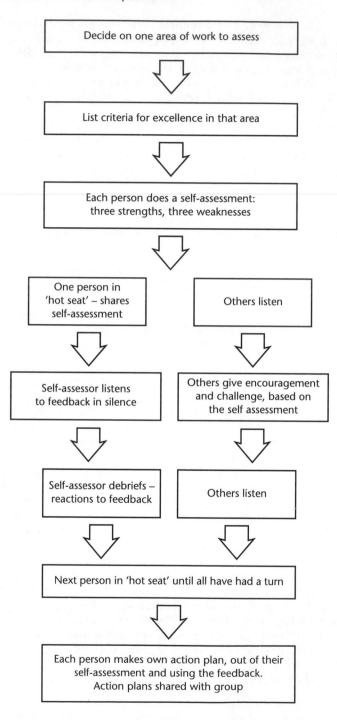

Figure 7.7　Steps in self and peer review

be unrealistic) and the denied self (our potential skills and gifted self which may have been suppressed in childhood and even in nurse training!) into the real self which is how we are and how we function within our socially constructed reality.

By 'peer' I mean those people who perceive themselves to be at an equal level in the organisational hierarchy, none of them having any managerial role over the other.

A structure for self and peer review in a clinical supervision group
As a group, decide on one aspect of your work which all group members have in common. In twos or threes, with a sheet of flip chart paper and felt pen, taking seven to ten minutes, make a list of phrases which would begin to offer answers to the following question: 'What abilities/skills/qualities/approaches/knowledge/attitudes/actions/results achieved make for a high standard of practice as far as (chosen area of your work) is concerned?' Be specific: rather than using one word, try to express each point in more than two words to clarify what you had in mind. For instance, rather than putting 'communication', put 'keeping colleagues informed about patient's changing needs'. Do not list descriptions of personality types; keep to specific abilities, etc. You do not have to agree with each other on each point: write all contributions onto the list, using one side of the paper only. At the end of the time, put all the lists together.

Working alone, each person makes an individual self assessment of their abilities. Out of all the criteria the group have produced, make a list of about 20 of the ones which you think are important. Reword them to fit your own words. Now pick out one of your strongest points from your list. If your confidence is having a bad day and you cannot think of a 'strength', then pick out something in which you think you are least hopeless! Then pick one of your weakest points from the list of criteria. If your humility is having a bad day and you cannot think of any 'weaknesses', then pick out one in which you are least brilliant!

Then identify a second strength and a second weakness, then a third of each. Ensure that your list has an equal number of strengths and weaknesses. It is important to strike this balance: many nurses are often too ready to be over-critical about themselves and list more weaknesses than strengths. Others are afraid to admit to weaknesses. Working in a group where each person is revealing a few can help get over this reticence. Ensure that you do not choose or interpret any criteria as being about your personality: this is an assessment of your expertise in the chosen area, not your personality. Write a sentence or two illustrating in concrete terms exactly how strong or weak you are in each particular criterion. Being vague is a common pitfall in this type of self-assessment. Vagueness can be a handy defence against challenging yourself to look at your abilities and weaknesses and making any concrete plans to change and develop.

The next stage is to set up the peer feedback in the group. Plan the order of taking turns to be in the 'hot seat'. Agree set amounts of time for each step: suggested timings for a group new to this approach are given in brackets.

More experienced groups may want to have longer. Taking your turn as the 'hot seat' person, tell the group your self-assessment (three minutes). Then listen silently to the feedback for the agreed length of time (allow one minute per person giving feedback, so five minutes if the clinical supervision group is five people plus facilitator). Write down the feedback, or have someone else do so. Silently evaluate each item as one of three categories: (1) Valid – yes, you agree; (2) Not valid – no, you disagree; or (3) Partially valid – perhaps there's something to think about.

Being silent can be very hard to do, since there is a tendency in most of us to explain or defend or to divert the process into a red herring discussion. If you find that the feedback is becoming overwhelming, with too much to take in, or is feeling unbalanced, with either too much cosiness or too much criticism, you can stop the process at any time. There is no purpose in continuing with something that is unhelpful.

When the feedback phase is over, you can speak by way of a debriefing (two minutes). You might want to say how you felt before, during or after the feedback, your reactions to specific points or to the overall experience, or top-of-the-head insights that came to you as a result of the process.

When you are one of the people giving feedback, listen carefully to the self-assessor and take brief notes of their self-assessment. Do not interrupt if there are any points you don't quite understand.

During the feedback phase, link every piece of feedback in some way to the self-assessment. Give encouraging feedback and some challenging nudges to enable the self-assessor to think about doing something differently or changing their approach. Some forms of words by way of triggers are suggested in the table. You will notice that most of the suggested forms of words are spoken in the first person: 'I think/feel', etc. This is important in this process. Speaking for yourself in this way acknowledges the subjectivity of your feedback, avoiding the pitfall of the pseudo-objectivity which can make feedback patronising or destructive. (See also Table 7.2.)

Comments about your colleague's personality are *not* part of this process: you are giving feedback about their abilities, skills or approach. Often, when doing this for the first time, groups tend to be anxious and, contrary to everyone's expectations, become too reassuring and cosy, contradicting the self-assessor's identification of weaknesses. Think of your challenges as gentle nudges to help the person in the 'hot seat' look at things another way and to stretch their existing skills and competencies to even greater heights. Allow the self-assessor to identify their weaknesses and encourage them to develop their abilities in these aspects, even if you think they are already skilled enough. Overall, try to keep a balance between the challenge and support that the group gives, and end on a positive note.

After each 'hot seat' exercise, note briefly the feedback that you gave and consider the extent to which each comment also applies to yourself.

Very occasionally, some groups can become gung-ho in giving too many challenges and not enough encouragement and support. We have found these are usually people who have recently learnt how to be challenging and want to over-use their new-found skill. Where the group members work together elsewhere than in the clinical supervision group, sometimes the

Table 7.2 Self and peer review: trigger phrases for giving feedback

Your personal reactions
– to your colleague's self-assessment, for instance:

'I liked most/least . . .',
'I agree/disagree with . . .',
'I notice you were more weighted towards the positive/negative',
'I am delighted/concerned that you said . . .',
'I'd like to encourage you to develop . . .'

Exaggerated hunches
Exaggerate own imagination, mental pictures or perceptions, even if no specific evidence, for instance:

'I imagine that in such-and-such a situation you might . . .',
'If let my imagination run riot, I can picture . . .',
'My worst fear is that you would . . .',
'My highest hope is that you would . . .',
'If I was your patient, I imagine that . . .'

Supportive challenging questions
– to give self-assessor something to think over, for instance:

'Do you really think . . . ?',
'When did you last actually . . . ?',
'What makes you think . . . ?',
'Are you aware . . . ?'
(The recipient of the feedback just receives these questions silently and records them to think over later)

Suggestions
– for instance, soft advice:

'Perhaps you could try . . .',
'One option/alternative/possibility could be . . .',
'You might try . . .',
'It might be useful to . . .',

or hard advice:
'It's very important that you . . . otherwise . . .',
'I strongly urge you to . . .'

Constructive challenging feedback
Comment on action/approach, not personality, for instance:

'I noticed that . . .',
'I think/don't think that . . .',
'I get the impression that . . .',
'It seems to me . . .',
'I'm concerned about . . .',
'I felt . . . when you . . .',
'I wonder if you really . . .',
'I noticed a contradiction between what you said about . . . and . . .'

Positive feedback
Comment on action/approach, not personality, for instance:

'I like the way you . . .',
'I valued/appreciated . . .',
'I felt pleased when you . . .',
'I support . . .',
'You have a right to . . .',
'I noticed one of your particular strengths is . . .'

feedback session can degenerate into giving vent to criticism and frustrations that belong to other occasions and settings, and should be dealt with outside the clinical supervision group.

When everyone has had a turn in the hot seat, each person takes time on their own to formulate a plan of action to develop not only each weakness, but also each strength (ten minutes). We find that people often tend to omit the latter in unstructured self-assessment. Be specific about what exactly you will do, when and how. Set realistic targets to prevent yourself slipping into patterns of negative thinking. Then get together again as a group and share action plans (five minutes). Make a note of others' plans so you can review next time how they got on.

Reciprocal clinical supervision in pairs

Some clinical supervision groups resolve the difficulty of ensuring each person has enough 'air time' by spending some time working in pairs. You divide the time you have available in two, and during the first clinical supervision session, one person in the pair is the supervisee and the other the clinical supervisor. Then at the end of the time, those who were clinical supervisors become supervisees and have their 'air time'. At changeover time, you can either swop roles in the pairs or rotate with other pairs: we find the latter works better, because nurses have a tendency to let the first supervisee run over time and take up the second person's 'air time'. It saves time to draw out the pairings on a board or sheet; for instance, in a group of six people, Session 1: A is supervisee, B is clinical supervisor; C is supervisee, D is clinical supervisor; E is supervisee, F is clinical supervisor. Session 2: B is supervisee, E is clinical supervisor; D is supervisee, A is clinical supervisor; F is supervisee, C is clinical supervisor.

This can be adapted to make training triads, whereby there is an observer with each pair. The observer's task is to sit back from the pair, out of the supervisee's line of vision and to note which supervisee and clinical supervisor skills are being used and to identify pitfalls. The observer then gives feedback at the end. It is important that the observer does not become involved in discussing the topic, however interested they are.

For the observers to get their turn as supervisees, there need to be three sessions, with changeovers in between.

For this structure to allow some in-depth reflection, each person needs to have at least 40 minutes as supervisee. The structure can, however, be used as a debriefing session of, say, ten minutes each, after some other group activity.

Some examples of clinical supervision group structures in action

Clinical supervision groups have adopted and adapted a variety of adaptations and combinations of these structures. The following examples highlight the need for close structuring and timing to ensure that clinical supervision does indeed take place and the group does avoid the rigour of clinical supervision by sliding into becoming a general chat, open-ended support or abstract discussion group.

For example, a peer group of six staff nurses from a number of different wards meet for two hours every six weeks. They each take a turn to facilitate the group, and the facilitator joins in with the activities. Each group member also receives one-to-one clinical supervision of one hour every six weeks, with a clinical supervisor who is not a group member. They have planned to experiment with various formats for group clinical supervision for the period of one year, and will decide then whether to continue with group clinical supervision and, if so, in what format or to have only one-to-one supervision, but more often. They have had three meetings so far. For the last two meetings, their format has been:

- settling: news, progress reports, practicalities (10 minutes)
- pairs: two-45 minute sessions. Session 1: A is supervisee, B is clinical supervisor; C is supervisee, D is clinical supervisor; E is supervisee, F is clinical supervisor. Session 2: B is supervisee, E is clinical supervisor; D is supervisee, A is clinical supervisor; F is supervisee, C is clinical supervisor
- completing: winding down, sharing action plans, planning next meeting (15 minutes)
- a total of 5 minutes is allowed for changeover time between the various activities.

They have decided to try the self and peer review format for the next two meetings, so this format will be:

- settling: news, progress reports, practicalities (10 minutes)
- self and peer review: listing criteria (10 minutes); self-assessment (10 minutes); each person in the 'hot seat' (3 minutes sharing self-assessment, 5 minutes feedback, 2 minutes debriefing) which is 6×10 minutes = 60 minutes
- completing: winding down, sharing action plans, reviewing how they felt about this structure, planning next meeting (15 minutes)
- a total of 10 minutes is allowed for changeover time between the various activities.

The next two meetings after that will have an adapted learning set structure:

- settling: news, progress reports, practicalities (10 minutes)
- learning set structure: one person (A) in the 'hot seat' for 45 minutes, reflecting in-depth with the help of other group members
- next person (B) in the 'hot seat' for 45 minutes, reflecting in depth with the help of other group members
- completing: winding down, sharing action plans, planning next meeting (15 minutes)
- a total of 5 minutes is allowed for changeover time between the various activities.

A group of mental health nurses, five people plus outside facilitator, meets for two and a half hours every month. Every third meeting is half an hour longer to allow for a review of the atmosphere of the group, the way they work together and the effectiveness of the clinical supervision that is taking place. Their format goes as follows:

- settling: news, progress reports, practicalities (10 minutes)
- learning set structure: one person (A) in the 'hot seat' for 45 minutes, reflecting in depth with the help of other group members
- pairs and triads: two 40-minute sessions. Session 1: B is clinical supervisor, C is supervisee, with the group facilitator as observer; D is clinical supervisor, E is supervisee, with A as observer. Session 2: B and C reverse roles and have A as observer; D and E reverse roles, with the group facilitator as observer. (Total: 50 minutes)

- completing: winding down, sharing action plans, planning next meeting (10 minutes)
- 5 minutes is allowed for changeover time between the various activities.

A group of eight nurse teachers in a university meet monthly for three and a half hours. Their format is:

- settling: news, progress reports, practicalities (10 minutes)
- learning set structure: the group divides into two groups of four, to take turns to be in the 'hot seat' for 45 minutes, reflecting in depth with the help of other group members
- 10 minutes is allowed for changeover times, hot drink, loo break
- completing: back together as a whole group, winding down, sharing action plans, planning next meeting (10 minutes).

You will see that for group clinical supervision to stand on its own, without being combined with one-to-one, a considerable amount of time must be allocated to the meetings to ensure each person has enough 'air time' in which to reflect in depth on their practice.

We emphasise that group clinical supervision is not an easy, quick or cheap option: quite the contrary. We do not usually recommend clinical supervision in groups for nurses without also having one-to-one: meeting the need for continuity and sufficient 'air time' is seldom possible. Creating a group of consistent membership, with the same people able to attend each time, is out of the question in most branches of nursing: it is just not possible to synchronise the availability of five or six people. It is seldom that cover for staff can be arranged to enable them to attend a clinical supervision group meeting of adequate length to allow each individual adequate 'air time' in which to reflect in depth. We examine in more detail the advantages and disadvantages of group clinical supervision as opposed to one-to-one in the next chapter.

If, however, group clinical supervision is possible and preferred we hope this chapter has been useful in clarifying a picture of group clinical supervision, and has provided enough pointers for a new group to start or for an established group to review whether or not its structure is effective.

Part III
Organising clinical supervision systems

8 ▷ Setting up clinical supervision

In this final chapter we wish to bring some of the themes of the book together to focus on the practicalities of setting up clinical supervision systems. We are concerned that conditions for effective implementation will fade under the competing pressures on both individuals and organisations. We want to reiterate the themes of the introductory chapters: the need to ensure a balance in implementing the principles of clinical supervision and, in so doing, to seek to diminish the adverse effects of resistant forces. Effective clinical supervision systems need to see a merging of practical endeavours from both those individuals on the ground who will be most directly involved in them, and those within the managerial and organisational structure who can help enshrine them in the fabric of the culture.

Conditions necessary for an effective clinical supervision relationship

Before we consider the options open to you in terms of delivery models or modes of clinical supervision, we want to place the relationship between supervisee and clinical supervisor at the centre of any strategy for developing any clinical supervision system. It is important to consider the conditions that need to apply for the working alliance to develop.

Unacknowledged fears of relationship can negatively influence the implementation of clinical supervision, creating the conditions for superficiality and resulting in a lack of support and rigour in clinical supervision. We suggest that seven conditions need to apply to give the opportunity for an effective relationship to develop: sufficient frequency of sessions to provide enough face-to-face time together; a long enough period of 'air time' at each meeting for the supervisee to be able to reflect in depth; continuity of clinical supervisor or group membership; a clear, mutually negotiated working contract; training in both supervisee and clinical supervisor skills and also in

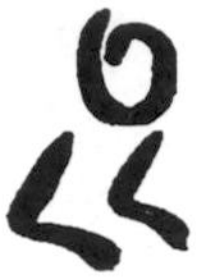

Frequent sessions – e.g. monthly

Individual 'air time' – e.g. one hour

Continuity of supervisor or group

Mutually negotiated contract;
including confidentiality

Training: supervisee, clinical
supervisor skills, group skills

Some choice of supervisor
and supervisee

Choice of mode

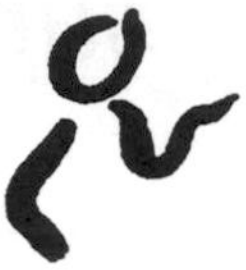

Figure 8.1   Conditions for an effective clinical supervision relationship

group skills where relevant; some mutual choice about clinical supervisor/ supervisee; choice of mode (one-to-one, triad or group) (see Figure 8.1).

There needs to be enough contact time structured into the delivery system for face-to-face contact between the supervisee and clinical supervisor so that a relationship and skills of clinical supervision can develop. Delivery systems that offer one hour three or four times a year are merely paying lip service to the concept of clinical supervision: there is no chance to get to know each other within the special context of clinical supervision and to build enough trust for effective in-depth reflection to take place. For instance, Johnson (1995), despite supporting the range of opportunities and merits of clinical supervision, goes on to advocate, from a management perspective, a minimum frequency of a mere two sessions a year. Admittedly this suggestion is only a minimum, but usually minimum standards become the depressing norm.

Having planned the time in, it needs to be protected by all concerned: management backup is needed to allow the supervisee to get away from the demands of the work setting, and supervisee and clinical supervisor need to give priority to punctuality, especially if travelling time has to be taken into account. Attendance is a crucial issue here: the relationship cannot happen if the people involved are not there. There can often be a vicious circle as far as this issue is concerned. At an individual level, someone who is not committed to clinical supervision is less likely to make the arrangements necessary to be able to turn up: their time management will be poor and they will not assert their need for cover from their colleagues or manager and will therefore always have the excuse of being too busy to attend on time or at all. At an organisational level, managers who are not committed to clinical supervision will not make explicit the expectation of attendance nor provide the backup resources to ensure that clinical work is covered in order to release staff. Ragged attendance means an unsatisfactory experience of clinical supervision, with further loss of commitment and so on, until the reality of clinical supervision disappears into thin air.

Another dimension of the time issue is 'air time', the time each individual supervisee has to reflect on their practice and the part they play in the quality of that practice, facilitated by the clinical supervisor or group. The supervisee needs blocks of reflection time of at least 45 continuous minutes in order to engage in facilitated in-depth reflection on their practice and on the part they play as a person in the quality of that practice. This is seldom available when the group mode of clinical supervision is chosen on its own: one-to-one offers more possibility of meeting this criterion. We recommend that one hour per month should be the target: this allows for a session to cover a review of progress and agenda-setting, 45 minutes in-depth reflection, and finally some action planning to be reviewed at the next session. In the consultation discussions prior to the publication of the UKCC (1996) position statement on clinical supervision, there was much agreement on this issue, although the paper did not include this figure. We get the impression that it is likely that the one hour per month rule of thumb will come into play much more in the near future. You will note that a system that offers one hour of one-to-one clinical supervision for three sessions a year pans out at 15 minutes per month on average, which is woefully inadequate. Likewise, we have come across a 'group clinical supervision' system where 11 people meet for one hour per month: this averages out at a maximum of four and a half minutes per person of 'air time' per month! We will explore in more detail the advantages of one-to-one and group clinical supervision later in the chapter.

Knowledge of the attachment needs of adults, touched on in Chapter 2, illustrates the need for continuity, reliability and establishing and maintaining boundaries. The supervisee needs to have the same person or people at each clinical supervision session, otherwise relationship building goes back to square one each time there is a change. This continuity is usually easy to maintain in one-to-one clinical supervision but many clinical supervision groups end up having variable composition because of difficulty in fixing dates suitable for all, the problem exacerbated the larger the group is. This is illustrated in the study by Butterworth *et al.* (1997), where the one clinical supervision group of five members was usually attended by only three of them each time. Continuity of venue should be attempted too, reducing the stress of getting there by knowledge of timings and routes, etc. The reliability of having the same person(s), who is/are committed to the process of clinical supervision, and can be punctual and settled enough to pay attention, is a vital part of building the relationship. The contract and boundaries of the relationship need to be mutually understood and accepted, clearly established, worked within and regularly reviewed, as we outlined in Chapter 3. This contract especially needs to include confidentiality, with very clear understanding of the conditions in which it could, in theory, be broken. It is important that the people involved have some chance to use their own wording for the contract, in order to ensure they fully understand each other and feel ownership of it.

Training in the skills of clinical supervision is usually essential. Indeed, in the study by Butterworth *et al.* (1997), they found this to be the principal 'hot issue' identified by those involved in the study, who emphasised the need for appropriate educational preparation for clinical supervisors. However, in our experience, training for supervisees is equally important and the most often overlooked. Only the most recently trained nurses have had significant training in reflective skills, and most nurses need some training in the skills we identified in Chapters 3 and 4. It could be argued that if all supervisees had enough understanding of the aims of clinical supervision, and were skilled enough at reflection and assertiveness, they could take charge of the clinical supervision sessions and train their clinical supervisors on the job, though this would take time and they may get a raw deal for the first few years. If we focus on the training needs of clinical supervisors: all research studies that we have found that look into the nurse/patient or teacher/learner communication skills of nurses have highlighted that non-directive skills are lacking across the board. Any clinical supervision system that assumes a body of staff have enough skills in the facilitation of another's reflection is likely to founder, even in fields where such skills are often assumed to be stock-in-trade, such as mental health nursing, health visiting and nurse education. Our experience in training workshops bears this out. An increasing number of nurses have also trained as counsellors or psychotherapists, but we find that this group often need training in incorporating more challenging and informative skills, and need to focus on the aims of improving practice, and of clearer boundaries as to the extent of probing into personal issues of supervisees. Another vital dimension to address, if group clinical supervision is being considered, is the area of group skills. We attempted to highlight in Chapter 7 that this option is not the easiest one, as is often mistakenly assumed: skills of group participation and supervisee and clinical supervisor skills are required by all involved, as well as group facilitator skills by the facilitator.

For staff to have ownership of a clinical supervision system and for getting a clinical supervision relationship off to a good start, there needs to be the maximum amount of choice of mode of clinical supervision and choice of clinical supervisor. Deciding whether to have one-to-one or group clinical supervision should be the choice of specific groups of staff themselves and, if possible, the individual should have the choice within the clinical supervision system that is set up. Different personalities benefit more from one or other of the modes and it can be detrimental to slot people into a form of clinical supervision which does not fit, when another could be more fruitful.

Having a real choice of who to see as clinical supervisor is essential to building a working alliance. Clinical supervision is inevitably a process in which self-disclosure needs to happen and a supervisee may not feel empowered or trusting enough with a clinical supervisor who has been allocated. Nurses often avoid the choice issue in case a clinical supervisor's feelings are hurt if they are not chosen, but the quality of clinical supervision and ultimately the quality of care must not be compromised because of this fear. If one person is consistently not being chosen, this may highlight issues which need to be addressed about them as clinical supervisor, whether these are to do with their individual abilities or qualities, or the position they hold in the organisation. Where people are employed expressly to do clinical supervision, there is a special problem about choice, but this can be overcome.

Some staff will not want to have this person as supervisor because they may be seen as too intimately connected to the immediate management structure, but may be willing to see another similar clinical supervisor in another hospital or locality, or arrange their own supervision with a peer colleague. Likewise, the clinical supervisor should have the choice about whether or not to work with a particular person. Membership of a clinical supervision group must be afforded the same attention. Allocation of members is unlikely to lead to success: members need to have some choice. When we emphasise choice, we realise that total free choice is impractical and, in some cases, undesirable. A choice of two or three clinical supervisors is preferable, or perhaps the freedom to express first and second choices from a list of possible clinical supervisors. As we stated in Chapter 3, we see this as an equal opportunities issue.

Developing clinical supervision as a distinct entity

The most common pitfall we see in the organisation of clinical supervision is to simply rename some other existing form of communication as 'clinical supervision'. This may be done unintentionally, from misunderstanding or mental blocks, but we have seen this done intentionally as a means of ticking off clinical supervision as 'done'. Staff and purchasers are becoming more alert to this practice and see it as inadequate.

Naturally enough, people will tend to view clinical supervision as being connected to the particular communication systems to which they themselves are most committed in their role within the organisation. As coordinators, many will want to combine clinical supervision with the familiar communication system, at the expense of protected time for the supervisee's in-depth reflection on practice. Indeed, you could dip in and out of this book and find elements which will help you to develop other systems, but be alert to the temptation to simply rename another type of communication as 'clinical supervision'. Senior managers who themselves have never experienced the supportive and developmental element of clinical supervision may not understand its nature and may see its introduction as a heaven-sent opportunity to improve or replace other communication systems which are not as effective as they might be.

Clinical supervision needs to be established, developed and protected as an entity in itself. The culture of the NHS at this time is too hierarchical and too anxious to enable creative combinations which truly allow for the principles of clinical supervision to be upheld. This culture affects not only the way a well-intentioned supervisor may set about clinical supervision, but the depth to which a supervisee may be able to make use of it. We need to use effectively and develop the other communication systems in their own right. Clinical supervision is not a replacement for any of these systems.

We have seen many such renamings of various communication systems as clinical supervision: 'clinical supervision' as child protection monitoring; 'clinical supervision' as a complaints procedure; 'clinical supervision' as Individual Performance Review; 'clinical supervision' as management by objectives;

Table 8.1 Emphasising the distinctive place of clinical supervision

	Management monitoring	*Support and development*
Clinical supervision is distinct from these other communication systems.	Complaints procedure Day-to-day monitoring of standards Disciplinary procedure	Ad hoc peer support Ad hoc support from manager Case conferences Clinical teaching

It should augment them.	Management by
	  objectives
		Consultation exercise for
		  developing strategy, policy

Clinical supervision should not be amalgamated with any of these systems.	Managers briefing staff
	Performance appraisal
	  (Individual
	  Performance Review)
		Debriefing sessions after
		  traumatic events
		Educational assessment
		In-service training and

Nor should it replace or undermine any of these important means of communication between staff.	Staff giving service
	  delivery information
	  to managers
	Team meetings
	Work hand-over meeting
		development
		Mentorship
		Occupational health backup
		Personal counselling
		Preceptorship
		Specialist clinical advice, e.g.
		  infection control; child
		  protection; HIV; hospital/
		  community liaison
		Staff support group

'clinical supervision' as a staff support group, and so on (see Table 8.1). In all cases, the unique blend of formative, restorative and normative functions that we describe in this book as being 'clinical supervision' are not possible. Again, we wish to reiterate that we do not view any of these systems as having less value than clinical supervision; they are just different. The fact that we devote a whole book to clinical supervision does not diminish the importance of these other systems, but you will need to look elsewhere for guidance about how to develop them.

As an example of this renaming, Valerie was the ward manager of a general medical ward, with 24 staff divided between three teams, each with a team leader. She already had in place a system of 'management by objectives', to which she was very committed. She was faced with a Trust directive that staff receive one hour per month of clinical supervision. As is common, no extra resources were made available to release staff and she felt anxious about getting the work done within the existing resources, so decided to rename her management-by-objectives system in the hope that that would cover it.

Her approach to management by objectives was a vertical cascade system: she met with each team leader for one regular hour a month, and each of them had a one-hour meeting with each individual member of her team, with the option of having additional meetings as necessary. These meetings were guided by a supervision form, devised by Valerie, which was completed after each meeting, copies kept by the supervisee, supervisor and one sent to Valerie. She decided the groundrule of confidentiality was unrealistic. The meetings comprised drawing up an agenda, with topics brought by the supervisee and then by the supervisor, then working through each topic in turn. The supervisor's responsibility was clarified as being to explore the extent to which managerial and team objectives were being met, and to receive an account of work done. Valerie herself had monthly meetings with the business manager, during which there was mutual briefing and the setting and reviewing of Valerie's objectives. She felt that the supervision system was going well, and when she asked staff they agreed. What they especially valued about it was the individual contact with their line manager, and knowing exactly where they stood and what they were supposed to be doing. She certainly felt as a manager that she was doing her best and was fulfilling the Trust directive. She then took up another post on another ward.

In this example, Valerie had already built a good management monitoring system and by renaming it, she felt she was providing 'clinical supervision': her business manager had a similar misconception. Subsequent events showed that this could be developed into a system which fulfilled more of the supportive and formative functions of clinical supervision, without displacing the 'management by objectives' approach.

Valerie left to take up another post. Her successor, Brian, was impressed with the system as a managerial supervision system but it appeared to him from the records of the sessions and from talking with staff that reflective practice did not figure highly. The UKCC (1996) guidelines had just been published and he was aware that the system was a managerial supervision system, not 'clinical supervision' in the sense described by the guidelines. His own previous experience of clinical supervision was more in line with the UKCC's position, and he had studied clinical supervision for a project during a management training course. He decided to change the system, with the aim of ensuring that staff had some protected time for in-depth reflection on practice, whilst retaining the effectiveness of the managerial system that Valerie had developed. He set up monthly supervision for himself, with another ward manager, Georgina, who he knew had been able to develop separate managerial and clinical supervision systems for her staff. He gained her cooperation in taking part in his project.

He changed the system as follows, with the intention to review it after six months:

- each member of staff received copies of some articles about clinical supervision, some guidelines and a 'bill of rights' for supervisees, a guide sheet for team leaders to distinguish between their roles as team leaders and clinical supervisors; some books were bought for the ward from funds donated by patients
- each of the team leaders have management meetings with Brian, at least monthly for at least half an hour AND have confidential clinical supervision sessions of one hour every two months, to focus on reflection on practice, with Georgina
- all team leaders continue to have meetings with each individual member of staff, in order to review team, organisational and individual objectives and receive an account of the work. The minimum standard is half an hour, once monthly, with the requirement to increase time and frequency

Table 8.2 Distinguishing between clinical supervision and management supervision

	Clinical supervision session	Management supervision meeting	IPR meeting	Disciplinary interview
Agenda setting	Agenda mostly defined by the supervisee. Clinical supervisor may highlight items arising from the content of sessions or about the way the working relationship is going	Agenda defined by manager and practitioner together	Agenda defined by IPR document, devised by manager, possibly with some input from practitioners	Agenda defined by manager
Confidentiality	Almost total, with exceptions of legal or professional ethics. Possibly a record of attendance dates and times. Record of content negotiated between practitioner and clinical supervisor, for their eyes only	Not necessarily confidential, but discretion used in passing on information about practitioner, e.g. to selected team members in order to ensure effective team functioning. May be recorded in manager's own notes and/or in personnel file	Not confidential, but discretion used in passing on information about practitioner. Copy of IPR document may be kept in manager's file and/or in personnel file	Not confidential, but discretion used in passing on information about practitioner. Recorded in manager's file and personnel file
Information giving and advice	Some information, advice, guidance offered to supplement the supervisee's own expertise, to help the supervisee see options available and make own informed decision	Information, advice and guidance given to direct the practitioner towards team and organisational objectives. Information given about policy directives	Information, advice and guidance given to direct the practitioner towards team and organisational objectives and training opportunities within the organisation	Information given about the disciplinary procedure and to direct towards improving the performance which is being challenged. Information about consequences of not improving

Challenging	Challenging technical mistakes, inadequate clinical standards, contribution to problems with team work, more personal issues such as unhelpful or self-defeating behaviour or attitude, blind spots, broken contracts. Based on evidence gained during the clinical supervision session	Challenging technical mistakes, inadequate clinical standards, contribution to problems with team work, lack of achieving pre-agreed objectives. Based on evidence gained/observed in any work situation	Challenging technical mistakes, inadequate clinical standards, contribution to problems with team work, lack of achieving pre-agreed objectives. Based on evidence gained/observed in any work situation	Challenging severe and/or repeated technical mistakes, inadequate clinical standards, contribution to problems with team work, lack of achieving pre-agreed objectives. Based on evidence gained/observed in any work situation
Support	Support for the supervisee as a person and encouragement given to help supervisee recognise and use own expertise and personal abilities towards developing their professional expertise. No practical help given outside sessions	Support and encouragement given to help supervisee recognise and use own expertise and personal abilities towards meeting specific team and organisational objectives. Practical help may be given outside the meeting	Support and encouragement given to help supervisee recognise and use own expertise and personal abilities towards meeting specific team and organisational objectives. Practical help may be given outside the meetings	Some support offered: often not a situation in which the practitioner can easily accept support from the person involved. Practical help may be given outside the meetings
Catalytic help	Enabling reflection on issues ultimately affecting practice, learning from experience, problem solving, pinpointing ways of dealing with difficult emotions, decision making and planning and reviewing application to practice	Manager elicits information from practitioner about work done and standards achieved. Enables problem solving on team and management issues	Manager elicits information from practitioner about standards achieved in the areas of practice outlined on the IPR document. Enabling overall performance review, problem solving, goal setting	Manager elicits information from practitioner about the issues under discussion. Enables goal setting

when either the staff member or the team leader has a concern, and the team leader is explicitly required to be available for ad hoc guidance when necessary. (Brian had discovered that staff were sometimes inappropriately saving up some technical concerns for their meeting rather than dealing with them at the time)

- each team member also has a clinical supervisor who is not her team leader (with an initial choice from the other team leaders on the ward or those from Georgina's), and they meet for one hour every two months for reflective clinical supervision, with a confidentiality contract
- records are kept of attendance at clinical supervision, but nothing is officially recorded about the content of sessions. Staff were advised to keep their own confidential record of their reflection during clinical supervision sessions and to select extracts to put in their professional portfolio.

This approach does not take any more time than the previous one, but Brian hopes that it will eventually progress to monthly clinical supervision. He was concerned that staff had not been able to get any training in the skills of clinical supervision, since his business manager could not be convinced that it was necessary, but he had a lot of goodwill from the staff and thought he would go ahead. Six months on, his staff evaluated the system as developing well: the first two sessions had been confusing as supervisees and clinical supervisors had struggled to adapt their use of the time from the management meetings they were used to. By the third session, the experiences of the clinical supervisors in their own clinical supervision sessions with Georgina were having an effect, giving them more of an idea of how to be clinical supervisors. Generally, staff were positive, and wished to increase the clinical supervision sessions to every six weeks.

This example illustrates the most common confusion that arises between clinical supervision and management supervision. Table 8.2 outlines some examples of differences between clinical supervision and management by objectives, IPR, and disciplinary interviews, in terms of what actually happens in the relationship during the meetings.

Need for managers to let go of control of clinical supervision

Throughout this book we have advocated that clinical supervision needs to be separate from managerial supervision in order that distinctions between use of 'power over' rather than 'power to' do not become blurred. As a manager, you personally may feel ready to distinguish between management and clinical supervision and may feel that you could hold distinct meetings with your staff to fulfil the separate functions. However, your staff are unlikely to be so ready, given the culture of nursing and the tensions within the NHS at present. In Parkinson's (1992) early study of the effectiveness of this combined supervision, nurse managers reported no difficulties in separating their managerial role from their advice and support role but did admit that they thought that some staff had difficulty responding to the latter. Their staff agreed, tending to see the potential disciplinary and control function as predominant.

Letting go of their personal involvement with the clinical supervision of their own staff will be difficult for many managers, who feel that they are committed to clinical supervision and combine these roles within the system they have already set up. In the early days of developing clinical supervision, many proactive, supportive and caring managers set up systems which they hoped might reflect support and professional development principles, and yet, by combining or confusing clinical supervision with forms of management supervision, they have unwittingly skewed these systems towards a mainly normative function.

The logistics as well as the ethics of combining the two would place an enormous strain on already depleted numbers of non-clinical managers. In Parkinson's (1992) study many managers did admit that they really did not have enough time to combine the roles due to an excess of competing demands from their other management responsibilities. Managers who have attended our courses have also reported that the amount of anxiety it causes them to hear of the uncertainties and vulnerabilities of large numbers of their staff is too much to expect of someone whose responsibility lies in managing the overall service. They find it a relief to articulate the impossibility of combining the role of an effective clinical supervisor with their diverse spread of functions, and begin to see their role as facilitators, enablers and sponsors of clinical supervision systems. These roles taken on by managers provide a crucial link between implementation in practice, and the structural acceptance and development of clinical supervision in the larger organisation.

Managerial supervision of practice remains a vital organisational function. The development of clinical supervision should not undermine the role of managers. Indeed, as a result of one pilot clinical supervision project in which we were involved as consultants, staff requested annual IPR with their manager, in addition to the clinical supervision, since they felt more equipped to use IPR constructively. This is in contrast to many other Trusts, where staff attend IPR sessions unwillingly or avoid them if possible. Other communication systems must continue alongside clinical supervision, such as continued access to child protection advisors, as directed in *Working Together Under the Children Act* (Department of Health 1991b)

The most frequent source of blocks to the progress of clinical supervision is undoubtedly concern over how it will be resourced. The costs of training, cascading training to others, coordinating a system and providing sufficient cover in the clinical areas both during training and in implementation of clinical supervision may be considered low priority in the present financial climate, and we acknowledge the difficulties managers are under. This factor presents very real dilemmas: the temptation is to provide a watered-down, homeopathic dose of clinical supervision in the hope that it will have an effect, when what is needed is regular IV infusions of the full-strength medication.

Compromising to the point of offering an ineffectual clinical supervision system because of resource difficulties may be a result of the more unconscious resistance alluded to in Chapter 2. Clinical supervision may be viewed as a challenge to the authority and control of management. As Swain (1995: 45) seems to be revealing, of herself and of her former manager colleagues, there is as much fear of loss of autonomy, power and authority

Table 8.3 Roles of people involved in setting up and maintaining a clinical supervision system

Senior manager	Unit, ward or team manager	Coordinator
• Be the sponsor of the clinical supervision system, not directly involved but providing management backup • Initiate the setting up of a clinical supervision system, if the initiative has not already come from staff themselves • Make a case for, win and manage a budget to cover costs • Be an advocate of clinical supervision within the political climate of the organisation and maintain the integrity of the system, resisting pressure from powerful elements within the organisation who misunderstand or wish to misapply clinical supervision • Provide backup resources to allow unit, ward or team managers to release staff from their work areas to attend clinical supervision, the working group or training sessions • Describe the clinical supervision system for inclusion in the organisation's portfolio for purchasers • Monitor and evaluate the system	• Initiate the setting up of a clinical supervision system if the initiative has not already come from the staff themselves or from elsewhere in the organisation • Train as a clinical supervisor and provide clinical supervision to members of other units, wards or teams (not your own) and possibly to peer colleagues at your grade • Enable staff to be released from their work to attend clinical supervision, the working group or training sessions • Continue to use and develop your day-to-day managerial supervision with your staff. Avoid the temptation to try to pass on your management problems to the clinical supervisor of any of your staff • Avoid the temptation to intrude on the confidentiality of your staff's clinical supervision by asking their clinical supervisor about it • Take on the role of coordinator if appropriate • Ensure that you receive and use your own clinical supervision to cover the whole range of your work, with someone who is not your line manager • Ensure that you have supervision of the clinical supervision that you provide, with someone who would not compromise the confidentiality of your supervisee	• Initiate the setting up of a clinical supervision system if the initiative has not already come from the staff themselves or from elsewhere in the organisation • Investigate the level of interest and expertise in clinical supervision among staff • Convene and facilitate a working group comprising people who are interested in clinical supervision, at various grades and as multidisciplinary as possible • If there are other similar working groups within the organisation liaise between them and share information • Provide or seek backup managerial sponsorship, so the working group can implement the strategy for setting up clinical supervision

in managers as there is in staff: 'We should not deceive ourselves; power, authority and the opportunity to influence as managers are heady potions. Having got them, it can be very difficult to let them go, or to have them taken away, as many nurse managers, side-lined by organisational change, will know.' However she goes on to remind us that many managers do desire to be supportive to staff and have often seen this aspect of their role marginalised by pressure of work. She suggests that their own anxiety and guilt may be assuaged by being able to sponsor real clinical supervision – that is, if their own envy and resentment of being unsupported themselves do not get in the way!

Roles of people involved in setting up and maintaining a clinical supervision system

We outline here the possible roles of the various people within the organisation who are involved in setting up and evaluating a clinical supervision system. (See Table 8.3.) Further guidance about strategy is provided later.

Business or senior manager

The senior manager's role as sponsor of the clinical supervision system involves providing the organisational backdrop while others take centre stage. This management backup role involves being an advocate for genuine clinical supervision within the political climate of the organisation, to establish and maintain the integrity of the system, resisting pressure from powerful elements within the organisation who misunderstand or wish to misapply clinical supervision. Inevitably, this requires you to make a case for, win and manage a budget to cover costs of training and backup resources to allow unit, ward or team managers to release staff from their work areas to attend working group, training and clinical supervision sessions. You will need a framework for calculating additional staffing resource needs.

Wanda calculates the time costs of a one-to-one system as follows: one-off during introduction of clinical supervision: working group time is 80 hours (eight people attending five two-hour meetings) and training time is six hours × the number of staff who will receive clinical supervision, plus 18 hours × the number of clinical supervisors to be trained. She takes the average hourly cost of staffing the unit and multiplies it by the hours taken to come up with a figure for clarifying the initial setting-up costs. Then she calculates the ongoing time costs: attending clinical supervision takes two and a half hours per month per member of staff receiving clinical supervision (the supervisee and clinical supervisor's time plus travelling time) and attending working group. Ongoing monthly average costs of the working group meeting every six months are 2.66 hours per month (8 × 2 hours × 2 divided by 12). She takes the average hourly staffing costs and multiplies by the ongoing costs to get a figure for the permanent increase in staffing resources required.

You could be involved in initiating the first steps in setting up a clinical supervision system, if the initiative has not already come from staff themselves and perhaps the initial coordination of the system. Ultimately, you will have the responsibility for ensuring that monitoring and evaluation of the clinical supervision system are carried out.

Yours is the task of educating the purchasers about the added value of a genuine clinical supervision system within your organisation's portfolio for purchasers. Cuts in management systems are being demanded by purchasers as management is seen as expensive: it is timely to insert your case for clinical supervision at times of management cuts, as purchasers are more likely to accept its cost and its increased necessity. Professionally there is an even greater need for clinical supervision at such a time, though it can be difficult to get across this quality issue if the people you are dealing with on the purchasing side do not have nursing backgrounds, as is usually the case. This is the setting to emphasise the normative function, how clinical supervision is the only formal system so far which provides a window through which one nurse can get an in-depth view of the professional knowledge, thinking processes and values behind the other nurse's practice and be in a position to offer acceptable support and influential guidance and, if necessary, bring serious concerns to light. Thus the safety, risk management and clinical effectiveness element can be highlighted. The detail and subtlety of how this is achieved is unlikely to be of interest given all the other priorities that have to be addressed at this level. To back up your case, you could cite the specific recommendations to purchasers and employers included in the UKCC's (1996) guidelines, the Department of Health's (1993a) *A Vision for the Future* document and especially the report of the evaluation study by Butterworth *et al.* (1997), of which the summary recommendations are shown in Table 8.4.

Table 8.4   Extract from recommendations by Butterworth *et al.* (1997: 4)

Trust Boards should ensure that business plans contain a strategy for the development of clinical supervision . . . This should address issues of allocated time and resources.

Purchasing authorities should seek evidence of clinical supervision . . . in providing services as confirmation of good quality practice.

Employers should recognise and capitalise on the benefits of clinical supervision . . . as it will form part of a human resource strategy that facilitates recruitment, retention and continuing professional development.

Staff must be given time for clinical supervision and a suitable location in which to carry it out.

Attention must be given to the preparation and education of clinical supervisors . . . Employers will need to attend to these needs through their own training resources or approach educational purchasing consortia for additional support.

The training and development of supervisors . . . must prepare them to deal with the wide range of content which will be presented to them, and ongoing support should be provided to enable their continuing work.

Unit, ward or team manager

We are aware that in many Trusts, particularly in the community, the nursing management structure has become so 'flattened', with layers being eradicated, that the same senior practitioners who need to be considered and trained for the role of clinical supervisor also have the additional responsibility for organising the entire setting up of local clinical supervision systems. Although they do not have management responsibilities as reflected in grading and pay, they have become a very cheap option for Trusts and have the enormous stress of having organisational development responsibilities grafted on to their practice caseloads and team leader roles. If you as reader are in this position we acknowledge the difficulties you are under. We offer some pointers to highlight which aspects of the setting up and development of a clinical supervision system may be especially pertinent to you.

If the initiative has not already come from junior staff or from elsewhere in the organisation, you may need to set the ball rolling. You may be required to take on the role of coordinator if appropriate. You also need to train in the skills of the clinical supervisor and provide clinical supervision to members of other units, wards or teams (not your own) and possibly to peer colleagues at your grade.

You need to make arrangements to enable your staff to be released from their work to attend clinical supervision, the working group or training sessions, and to make a case to your business manager for resources to be allocated to provide increased staff cover.

As the team, ward or unit manager, you need to continue to use and develop your day-to-day managerial supervision with your staff. Avoid the temptation to try to pass on your management problems to the clinical supervisor of any of your staff. You need to monitor whether or not your staff are actually attending and find out the reasons if they do not get to the clinical supervision sessions, but avoid the temptation to intrude on the confidentiality of your staff's clinical supervision by asking their clinical supervisor about the content.

It is important that you ensure that you receive and use your own clinical supervision to cover the whole range of your work, with someone who is not your line manager. You may wish to combine this with supervision of the clinical supervision that you provide, but you need to be alert to the need to keep confidential the content of the work you do with your supervisees, so it is preferable that your own clinical supervisor does not know your supervisees.

Coordinator

Who the coordinator of a clinical supervision system is varies: it might be a senior manager, team manager or senior practitioner. If you are taking on the coordination of a system, you need to set your sights realistically by designing a process which you feel you can handle, which seeks to meet the clinical supervision needs of an appropriate number of staff, whether a small team of four, or all nurses within a whole Trust.

Table 8.5   Guidelines for the introduction of clinical supervision: a summary

---

1 Before introducing clinical supervision, its purpose should be discussed and clearly defined. This definition should be informed by a theoretical understanding of the role and function of supervision and, equally, by a practical understanding of the circumstances and needs of the unit and its staff
2 All staff should be involved in the process of planning and introducing a system of clinical supervision
3 Careful consideration should be given to the qualifications, skills and experience required of supervisors, and to their ability to meet the individual needs of supervisees
4 All supervisors should be given opportunities to receive training and learn the skills that are needed to provide supervision that is both constructive and supportive. Those who receive supervision should have similar opportunities to learn about their role as supervisees
5 All supervisors should also receive supervision, in order to monitor and develop the quality of supervision they provide
6 Supervision should be available to all practitioners, regardless of seniority
7 The content of supervision should be carefully defined, with boundaries agreed about what is and what is not to be dealt with in supervision time. The processes to be supervised should also be made clear
8 The relationship between supervisor and supervisee should be formally constituted. Groundrules should be negotiated and agreed
9 It is essential that clinical supervision is monitored and evaluated. Supervisees and supervisors should play an equal part in these procedures
10 Individual units need the support of their employing authority to implement and maintain a system of clinical supervision

---

Source: Extracted from Kohner (1994).

You may need to be the person who initiates the setting up of a clinical supervision system if the initiative has not already come from elsewhere in the organisation. The type of system you set up needs to be appropriate to the numbers and needs of the staff involved. Guidelines about developing a strategy are summarised in Figure 8.2 (p. 217) and outlined next.

Strategy for implementing clinical supervision

Few specific guidelines exist about how to set up and maintain a clinical supervision system.

General principles are offered by Kohner (1994), as shown in Table 8.5, and the UKCC's (1996) six key statements mirror some of these. Swain (1995) suggests that managers address four main issues, an approach which mirrors good management practice in determining and planning for health needs of clients: (1) the search for health needs of staff; (2) stimulating an awareness of health needs; (3) the influence of policies affecting health (of staff); and (4) the facilitation of health-enhancing activities. We have attempted to incorporate the main principles identified by Kohner (1994), the UKCC (1996)

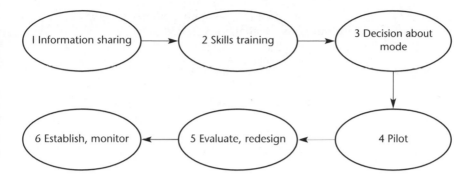

Figure 8.2 Strategy for implementing clinical supervision

and Swain (1995) into a practical six-stage framework for setting up and maintaining a clinical supervision system.

1 *Information sharing*

Investigate the level of interest and expertise in clinical supervision among staff. If the numbers of staff within your remit are too great for all to attend meetings for information sharing and discussion, convene and facilitate a working group comprising people who are interested in clinical supervision, at various grades and as multidisciplinary as possible, and include especially anyone with experience of clinical supervision. Those who have had experience of clinical supervision in previous posts or those who are trained as counsellors, and those who have studied clinical supervision during basic nurse or postgraduate training courses are valuable people to have on board. If there are other similar working groups within the organisation, in whatever discipline, liaise between them and share information. The medically allied professions, such as physiotherapy, occupational therapy, speech and language therapy and so on seem also to be interested in developing non-managerial clinical supervision and we have found that it is very fruitful to share information, training and, in some cases, a clinical supervision system, between the professions.

Encourage working group members to share books and journal articles on clinical supervision that they find useful for understanding and potentially for implementing clinical supervision, avoiding those which baffle or seem written for the sake of the author's academic CV rather than the practitioner. Focus your discussions on gaining enough understanding to begin to embark on a clinical supervision system, rather than aiming to understand everything about clinical supervision. There comes a point at which you cannot really understand any more unless you accept the uncertainty and just do it. We find that a pitfall of such working groups is to continue theoretical discussions beyond their usefulness, because of not wanting to face the discomfort of taking the leap into actually doing it. Indeed, some working groups have slid into becoming what they name clinical supervision groups but are actually continuing as avoidant discussion groups.

2   Skills training

Practical training in the skills of being a supervisee and a clinical supervisor are necessary and we have discussed the reasons in Chapters 2 to 7. If your remit is to cover numbers of staff larger than, say, 12, this can be done by buying in an outside education and training consultant, as it will be more cost-effective than sending so many people to outside courses. It also has the advantage that the courses can be tailor-made for your staff and you have the chance to monitor the content and the standard of training. If you get the cooperation of the training or human resources department, a rolling programme of skills training courses could be set up to meet the training needs of new staff in your Trust and also to generate income by selling places to nearby Trusts. Multidisciplinary training offers more flexibility and can be very useful, provided that the other professions are committed to using a non-managerial model of clinical supervision: we find this in MAPs (medically allied professions) but not in social work, for instance. Although nurses are usually reticent to begin with, they value the experience of learning clinical supervision skills with other professionals once they have tried it. Multidisciplinary skills training can help to focus on the skills of the interaction rather the nursing content, which is their purpose.

Sending selected people on external training courses is useful if only a few are to be receiving skills training at a time. Look outside your own immediate discipline for skills courses: provided the setting of the skills building is in non-managerial clinical supervision, the discipline is almost irrelevant. Look for courses that offer practice in skills building, which requires groups of 20 or under and a facilitative teaching style rather than lecture or seminar format. Beware of universities and colleges who are also under great financial pressures to get 'bums on seats' and earn money from courses with large groups, in which practical skills training is impossible. There may of course be some very good training available via these sources, but research them carefully. The time for conference-style information sharing on clinical supervision has probably passed since enough has been written about it, so it is more cost-effective for staff to share information between themselves as in Stage 1 of this framework.

Using self-training triads can be a cost-effective, though slow method of skills training. In this method, three people meet at least monthly for three and a half hours. They take turns to be supervisee, clinical supervisor and observer. After each (real, not role played) clinical supervision session of one hour, the observer gives feedback to both the supervisee and the clinical supervisor on the skills they used and the pitfalls they fell into in the session. The recipients of the feedback take notes and think over the feedback in between sessions. If this is the chosen method, it is useful during the 'information sharing' stage of this strategy to compile a lengthy checklist of skills and pitfalls of the supervisee and clinical supervisor. Observers in the triads then have a common framework from which to give feedback. Two

Table 8.6 Modes of clinical supervision

Pairs
- One-to-one with supervisor more experienced in the same field as the supervisee, not line manager, but in the same locality
- One-to-one with supervisor more experienced in the same field as the supervisee, not line manager, and in a different locality
- One-to-one with supervisor who is also line manager but has separate clinical supervision sessions, distinct from management role (not a recommended option)
- One-to-one with supervisor who has specialist expertise within supervisee's own field (e.g. child protection, HIV)
- One-to-one with supervisor from another discipline (e.g. clinical psychology) but supervisee has access to someone in own speciality for ad hoc sessions as necessary
- One-to-one with peer colleague, reciprocal in pairs
- One-to-one with peer colleague, in circular arrangement: A supervises. B who supervises C who supervises D who supervises A

Triads
- One-to-one, with a third person observing the supervisor, with a coaching role to enable supervisee and supervisor to develop skills

Groups
- Group with peer colleagues within the same discipline, led by supervisor who is more experienced in the same field of the supervisees and has group facilitation skills too
- Group with peer colleagues within the same discipline, led by supervisor who has specialist expertise within supervisee's own field (e.g. child protection, HIV) and has group facilitation skills too
- Group with peer colleagues of mixed disciplines, led by supervisor who has group facilitation skills
- Group with peer colleagues of same discipline, led in turn by group members
- Group with peer colleagues of mixed disciplines, led in turn by group members

essential groundrules are: that the observer stays absolutely silent throughout the session, sitting back out of eye contact; second, that the observer does not comment upon the content of the session, except to illustrate an example of a skill or pitfall, and definitely does not give any last minute advice, however tempting.

3 Decision about mode and structure

The next step is to decide as a working group on a mode of clinical supervision which is appropriate to you and your setting, having consulted any colleagues whom you are deemed to represent. The options are as outlined in Table 8.6.

Ensure that all clinical supervisors are included as supervisees in your structure. It is vital that they receive as well as give clinical supervision in order to build their understanding of the nature of the clinical supervision process and especially to enable them to deal with the added stress of being a clinical supervisor. Butterworth *et al.* (1997) showed that supervisors who

Table 8.7 Pros and cons of one-to-one clinical supervision as compared to group

Advantages	Disadvantages
More practical, easier to arrange mutually convenient times	Can be too intense a setting for supervisees who are not used to and afraid of self-disclosure
Supervisee more likely to get an appropriate amount of 'air time' in which to be able to reflect in depth	The choice issue is more critical: there must be some choice for the supervisee as to who to have as clinical supervisor. This is difficult if someone has been appointed to do clinical supervision. Even where there is choice, some nurses may choose someone in order not to hurt their feelings about not being chosen, rather than out of genuine preference, which gets the clinical supervision relationship off to a wobbly start. The supervisee may choose someone as an easy option, who they know will not challenge them. It being a one-to-one situation, there is no one else to do the challenging
Self-disclosure can be less frightening for more introvert individuals than in group situation	
More continuity, the same clinical supervisor each time	
May be preferred by individuals who have had bad previous experiences in learning groups	
Gives more of a sense of being listened to as an individual, cared for by the organisation	
The working alliance, the clinical supervision relationship, can develop more deeply more quickly	No one else there to referee if there is an argument or to dilute the effect of a personality clash
	Supervisee gets the perspective of only one other person

themselves did not receive clinical supervision were significantly more stressed than those who did receive it.

In choosing a mode, you need carefully to consider the pros and cons of each and to decide according to your priorities and needs. The advantages of one-to-one clinical supervision (Table 8.7) over group is that it is more practical, and it is easier to arrange mutually convenient times. This means that there is more continuity than is usual in group clinical supervision, since you are with the same clinical supervisor each time. The other main factor to take into account is that the supervisee is more likely to get an appropriate amount of 'air time' in which to be able to reflect in depth.

One-to-one clinical supervision may suit certain personality types: for more introvert individuals self-disclosure can be less frightening than in a group situation, or may be preferred by individuals who have had bad previous experiences in groups. This mode can give more of a sense of being listened to as an individual, of being cared for by the organisation. The working alliance, the clinical supervision relationship, can develop more deeply more quickly when there is only one person to get to know.

One of the main disadvantages for some people is that it can be too intense a setting for supervisees who are not used to and are afraid of self-disclosure. It may feel more like a counselling setting, especially uncomfortable if the supervisee has had bad experiences of counselling-type situations in the past.

The choice issue is very critical: there must be some choice for the supervisee as to who to have as clinical supervisor. This is difficult if someone has been appointed to do clinical supervision. Even where there is choice, some nurses may choose someone in order not to hurt their feelings about not being chosen, rather than out of genuine preference, which gets the clinical supervision relationship off to a wobbly start. The supervisee may choose someone as an easy option, who they know will not challenge them. It being a one-to-one situation, there is no-one else to do the challenging if that one person colludes.

If there is a disagreement or even an argument, there is no one else there to referee or to dilute the effect of a personality clash. The supervisee may feel trapped, working with someone with whom they cannot relate and they may not be assertive enough to make alternative arrangements. Lastly, one disadvantage is that the supervisee gets the perspective of only one other person on the issues brought to the session.

The advantages and pitfalls of coaching triads have been covered in the section on training. Three-way triads function as a small group and most of the issues and methods applying to group clinical supervision apply here.

Moving on to group clinical supervision (Table 8.8), we strongly caution you to consider carefully the criteria which need to be thought through before embarking on the group model of clinical supervision. We find that the group model is often chosen because it might appear, incorrectly, to be more time- and cost-effective than one-to-one: one clinical supervisor can 'do' five supervisees at once. Group clinical supervision is diluted and ineffectual when this is the only criterion for choosing this model. Other criteria need to be considered: here we will highlight some disadvantages in choosing clinical supervision, as they are often underestimated.

If the mistaken criterion of 'one clinical supervisor can do five supervisees at once' is applied, then each supervisee will get less than one fifth of the 'air time' that she would have received if she had been having one-to-one. For example, if a clinical supervision group of five people and one group facilitator meets for one hour every month, then each group member gets ten minutes of air time per session: this scanty amount of time pays only lip service to the aim of 'in-depth reflection' that is intended in clinical supervision (this timing allows for five minutes to settle in together as a group and five minutes to wind down and make plans for the next meeting). Many of the complicated issues that supervisees would want to bring to clinical supervision would take ten minutes or more just to explain to a group, there being no time for reflection at all. Some groups have a system of taking turns to be the supervisee: each week, one person has the whole 50 minutes to present an issue to the group and receive clinical supervision from them. This, however, means that each member of a group of five only receives clinical supervision once every five months, which is also woefully inadequate if this is not combined with one-to-one sessions as well.

If clinical supervision in a group is to provide sufficient 'air time', then many would consider that it is time-consuming rather than time-effective in comparison to one-to-one. Another factor to take into account is the time

Table 8.8 Pros and cons of group clinical supervision as compared to one-to-one

Advantages	Disadvantages
Setting for pooling of professional knowledge and expertise, by getting an insight into how individual group members manage their relationship as individuals with their practice	Time-consuming for each person to have adequate 'air time' and additional time needed for group dynamics
	In reality, individuals often get scanty amounts of 'air time'
Self-disclosure can be less frightening for more extrovert individuals than in a one-to-one situation	High level of skills needed: participants need supervisee skills *and* clinical supervisor *and* group participation skills; facilitator needs clinical supervisor skills *and* group facilitation skills
May be preferred by individuals who have had good previous experiences in learning groups	
Builds a sense of belonging to the team or organisation	Self-disclosure can be more frightening for more introvert individuals or those who have had bad previous experiences in learning groups
Reduces isolation and enhances feeling of being supported by the organisation: especially useful for practitioners who work on their own	Easier for non-committed individuals to 'hide' and say very little
	More difficult to arrange times for sessions which are convenient for all
Learning, changing and application to practice can be enhanced by the support and challenge of a group; the supervisee gets a variety of perspectives	Difficult to get continuity, since different people attending each time therefore less trust, less of a sense of a working alliance in which to reflect in depth
Group dynamics can be exciting and stimulating if all group members are very committed and skilled	More likely to slide into becoming a session for chat, general discussion, support or professional information updating rather than focusing on each individual's in-depth reflection
	Group dynamics can go wrong, and sabotage everyone's clinical supervision

needed to build and maintain positive group dynamics and to deal with the likely group dynamics problems that will arise from time to time. So, our group of five would need to meet for a whole day each month to allow enough time for five people to have one hour each, and to have settling time at the beginning, breaks and winding down time at the end. While we have found one group of managers able to make this time commitment, we have not yet come across any groups of practitioners who have been able to do this.

Receiving clinical supervision in a group setting will not suit every nurse's personality. Self-disclosure in a group can be more frightening for more introvert individuals than in a one-to-one situation. Dealing with the inevitable conflicts that arise in ongoing groups can be too scary for such nurses.

Some nurses have had bad experiences in groups and this has negatively coloured their expectations of the value of groups as a learning environment, even those with the most extrovert personalities. Others not committed to clinical supervision might choose a group mode in order more easily to hide and just go through the motions of participation.

Another crucial disadvantage of clinical supervision in a group rather than one-to-one is that it requires more skills. Participants require not only supervisee skills, but also clinical supervisor and group participation skills. The facilitator needs group facilitation skills as well as clinical supervisor skills. Finding or training people to possess these skills can be especially problematic when setting up clinical supervision from scratch, with few or no staff having had any previous experience of it.

Another practical disadvantage is that it can be more difficult to arrange times for sessions which are convenient for all. Usually this results in a lack of consistency in attendance, which not only exacerbates the practical problem of lack of 'air time', but also interferes with the consistency that is required for enough trust to be built up to enable in-depth rather than superficial reflection, and can make the dynamics of the group difficult. Varied group composition usually results in less cohesion and motivation to attend and the group can peter out.

Lastly, the group dynamics can go wrong and thereby reduce the effectiveness of the clinical supervision that each person receives. For instance, one member can sabotage the others' clinical supervision if, say, they are antagonistic towards clinical supervision or towards another person in the group. One group member who has difficulty in disclosing their own difficulties can hold back the development of safety in the group, so others will be reluctant to share anything significant and therefore the level of reflection that goes on in the group is superficial.

However, there are some definite advantages to choosing group rather than one-to-one clinical supervision. These relate to the potential for greater sharing of expertise, belonging, support and energy. The group can provide a setting for pooling of professional knowledge and expertise. This can work well if group members can contribute different perspectives from different professional experiences, such as mixing newly qualified practitioners with very experienced ones. The experienced practitioners can be brought up to date with recent approaches and the new practitioners can learn from the real-life experiences of the others. You might wish to have a mix of experiences from different branches of nursing.

You may choose to have clinical supervision in a group in order to build a sense of belonging. Some groups work well with the members being part of one team, and the spin-off from giving and receiving clinical supervision together is the team-building effect. Brown and Bourne (1996) describe this effect in social work teams. The group could be made up of people from different teams within a hospital or locality, and this can build a sense of belonging within a wider sector of the organisation. Group clinical supervision can be especially useful for practitioners who work alone a lot, reducing isolation and enhancing a feeling of being supported by the organisation.

Clinical supervision in a group setting may be preferred by nurses whose personality suits working in groups. Self-disclosure in a group can be less frightening for more extrovert individuals who might be more scared by being closeted alone in a room with one other person. Previous positive experiences of group work might lead even the quietest nurses to prefer group clinical supervision.

Tangible changes in practice can be more likely to occur in an effective clinical supervision group than in one-to-one clinical supervision. The challenge of a group can help the individual to accept difficult realities and get through defensiveness that might otherwise have led to the supervisee to dismiss a solo clinical supervisor's challenge. The support of the group can help the individual to have the courage to carry out difficult changes.

The dynamics of a clinical supervision group can be exciting and stimulating if all group members are very committed and have the necessary skills. The stimulation of being challenged by a supportive group can stretch and strengthen each member's reflection on their practice and can enhance their motivation for clinical supervision and for developing their practice.

If you choose a group mode of clinical supervision, then there is the decision to be made about whether or not to have an outside facilitator or to take turns to facilitate the group. Some options for an outside facilitator are:

- from another discipline (e.g. clinical psychology) or another speciality within nursing
- person appointed to a post in which the job role includes being a clinical supervisor, e.g. professional development workers, practice development nurses
- has specialist expertise within supervisee's own field (e.g. child protection, HIV), but content of clinical supervision session can include any other topics the supervisee wishes to bring
- senior who is not the group members' line manager, e.g. manager of another group or unit
- colleague at peer level who belongs to another clinical supervision group.

In other clinical supervision groups, members take turns to be the group facilitator. There are advantages and disadvantages in having an outside group facilitator or being peer-facilitated, summarised in Table 8.9.

There are two further decisions to be made about the organisational structure of the delivery system of clinical supervision: whether or not it is to be compulsory to attend, and second what records should be kept. One of the main problems arising from making attendance compulsory is that it may raise resistance, exaggerating the fears of clinical supervision being a management tool. Second, few Trusts have yet developed such a smoothly running system that appropriate training and genuine choice of supervisor exists, and it would be unreasonable to force someone into a clinical supervision relationship with an inappropriate clinical supervisor. On the other hand, the problems of having a voluntary system include the fact that probably the staff most needing professional development will not volunteer. When some then face disciplinary proceedings about instances of poor practice, they are likely to be required to attend clinical supervision in the future. As Dimond (1997a) points out, 'Nothing would render clinical supervision more infamous and unacceptable [than] for it to be seen as part of the disciplinary process'. We recommend a compromise that for the duration of the pilot

Table 8.9   Advantages and disadvantages of having an outside or peer group facilitator

Outside group facilitator

Advantages	Disadvantages
May be more skilled at group facilitation	Payment usually needed
Has more authority, easier to challenge negative group processes	Has to get own clinical supervision elsewhere
People not experienced at clinical supervision may find it useful to learn from the group facilitator's modelling	Group may be dependent on group facilitator, invest her with too much authority
Especially useful with group members not used to collaborative work and self-disclosure in groups	Group members do not learn how to facilitate groups
Especially useful when there are interpersonal tensions already existing between members of the group	

Group members take turns to facilitate the group

Advantages	Disadvantages
No payment needed	Has less authority, can be more difficult to challenge negative group processes
Group members learn how to facilitate groups	
Some group members may find it easier to collaborate and self-disclose in the group	May not have enough skill in group facilitation to deal with the difficulties arising in the group
Especially useful when group members are experienced at clinical supervision and/or collaborating and self-disclosing in groups	
Group members may have more commitment to making the group work well, owning the process	May be a tendency to avoid taking a directive role

project, attendance is voluntary. Then after a date agreed by the working group, all new contracts of employment could include compulsory attendance, provided there is real opportunity for some choice of supervisor and for training. Any staff applying for promotion would be required to show evidence of attendance and a brief statement from the clinical supervisor or group to the effect that commitment to the process had been displayed (without revealing anything about the content). In some Trusts, staff have to attend clinical supervision in their own time, during lunch breaks or outside working hours, because there is no management sponsorship to provide the necessary cover. In these cases, the Trusts give up their right to make attendance compulsory.

As far as records are concerned, the same legal principles apply as with any other records. The patient has a right of access to any records which bear their name. The employer has a right to any records that are written about sessions that take place during work time, and can use them in disciplinary proceedings. If attendance is compulsory as part of an explicitly agreed employment contract, the employer has a right of access to records of attendance.

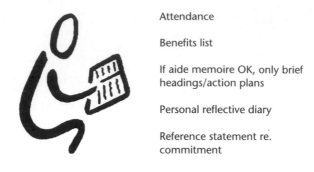

Attendance

Benefits list

If aide memoire OK, only brief headings/action plans

Personal reflective diary

Reference statement re. commitment

Figure 8.3 Possible records of clinical supervision

Any employer which invests resources into a clinical supervision systems also has a right to a record which indicates the benefits or otherwise of clinical supervision. As Dimond (1997b) points out, in theory, courts can subpoena witnesses to bring any relevant records to court, including personal diaries, though this is unlikely and such personal records hold little weight.

Therefore, we recommend the following records of clinical supervision be kept, without mentioning any patient's name (see also Figure 8.3):

- attendance date and time
- brief list of benefits written by the supervisee, say yearly
- if the supervisee agrees to an aide memoire being kept, we suggest that you write only general topic headings such as 'case review; stress management; time management; team work', etc. and possibly some specific action plans. What is written needs to be agreed by the supervisee
- personal reflective diary, written on supervisee's own stationery and kept confidential to herself and in own home
- brief statement by clinical supervisor or group by way of a reference for promotion, about level of commitment to the process of clinical supervision

4   Pilot

The next stage is to try out the mode you have chosen. Identify criteria for success by asking staff to pinpoint answers to these questions: 'Imagine that at the end of this pilot you definitely considered it a success. How would you know that it was a success? What exactly would be happening that would tell you it was a success?' Ensure that participants have had at least three clinical supervision meetings before you stop to evaluate, preferably six, in order to give the relationship a chance to begin to be established.

5   Evaluate, redesign

Attempts to evaluate clinical supervision systems are notoriously difficult. As Butterworth (1996: 96) suggests, 'The ideal research answers will, of course, be those in which clinical supervision is shown to have an impact on patient outcome', but he has not yet been able to devise such an evaluation tool. He goes on to state that at this early stage, a more measured and wide-ranging approach is likely to produce more satisfactory and reliable results. The 'feel-good' factor for staff may well be central to high standard performance, and recent encouragement to care for and develop the workforce has some merit.

(p. 96)

This qualitative dimension may be difficult to capture but is likely to be more important than the alternative quantitative measures. The entire project could be set up as an action research project following guidelines suggested by Hart and Bond (1993). Specific groups of staff could set up a cooperative enquiry, using models suggested by Reason (1988). Focus groups facilitated by an impartial outsider could be used to evaluate staff responses to the pilot.

Butterworth (1996) presents a range of tools and research methods linked to potential benefits to be accrued in each of Proctor's (1986) three key functional areas – for instance, existing mechanisms of sickness rates, absence, recruitment and retention and complaints could be used to audit staff satisfaction in the normative dimension as well as including client responses concerning satisfaction, complaints and health gain. Stress and burn-out scales could be used to evaluate the support (restorative) sphere, whilst the learning profiles and clinical skills development could be used to assess their professional development in the formative component. Structured or unstructured one-to-one interviews from an outside researcher could be used to evaluate all three functional areas. The 'rich pictures' (Checkland 1970) approach could be used to feed back the information collected.

We would like to return to anecdotal evidence to suggest improved 'feel-good' factors in examples of effective clinical supervision. Model 2 in Swain's (1995: 56) overview of the monitoring and impact of supervision said: 'The difference is somehow tangible; there is a sense of more openness and a positive approach', and, in Model 3: 'the practitioner is more confident and assertive, begins to decide objectives, begins to see goals and progress. It is easy to think that nothing has happened, as often the milestones reached are only small. However sickness rates have been seen to drop while in supervision, and to rise for one recently qualified practitioner when supervision had to stop'. In Parkinson's (1992: 52) study the 'managers . . . noted the beneficial effects on safe practice which had been achieved particularly in terms of working more openly with families, record keeping and better report writing. One manager also thought a large number of staff felt safer in their work'. Clearly anecdotal evidence such as this is inadequate by itself but we hear a similar range of positive responses in early reviews of systems. There is a long way to go before links to staff satisfaction, increased competence and confidence may be translated into demonstrable benefits for clients, but meanwhile anecdotal evidence has its place.

6 Establish and monitor

The methods you choose to evaluate your pilot scheme will depend on the scale of your project and will throw up any need for redesigning your clinical supervision system. When you have clarified and implemented this redesign, your clinical supervision system is underway and you need to adapt some of your evaluation methods to use as monitoring tools. The all-important sponsorship by a senior manager of the ongoing clinical supervision system needs to continue to be high profile and explicit in its support for the staff, as they continue to refine and develop their clinical supervision.

Looking to the future

Health care is now being provided in a mixed-economy, increasingly diverse system, in which the fragmentation of the profession of nursing is rapidly escalating. Nurses are being employed in a wide variety of settings in organisations which require their expertise but provide no nursing management monitoring backup. These include private companies with nursing homes, various types of organisations running group homes for people in the community with disabilities, social services, GP practices and voluntary organisations as well as the emergence of self-employed, freelance practitioners. Concern is increasing for these isolated practitioners, with increasing emphasis being placed on the need for clinical supervision, for instance, as shown by the special learning resources made available to practice nurses by the Department of Health (1996a).

Even within NHS Trusts, unidisciplinary management structures are considered too expensive and practitioners are increasingly working in multi-disciplinary teams with little or no specifically nursing management supervision. The argument about whether clinical supervision should be managerial or non-managerial is irrelevant to many nurses already, since they have no nursing manager who could do it. If present trends continue, there will be even fewer nursing managers. In the midst of all this fragmentation, the issue for the individual will be more about creating a professional and psychological secure base within which to receive support and understanding, and to reflect in depth on practice and on the part played as an individual in the quality of that practice, in so doing taking part in professional, rather than managerial, monitoring.

Nursing is increasingly likely to become a profession of autonomous practitioners who, like counsellors and psychotherapists, will become responsible for finding their own professional support and monitoring. In the introduction we quoted Alison Norman's concern that good ideas so often get lost in our profession. She goes on to say that 'to get [clinical supervision] wrong would be a tragedy for nursing and health visiting' (Norman 1995: 25).

Writing a book is one way of emphasising the importance of trying to get clinical supervision right for the profession of nursing, the individuals within it and their patients and clients, of making a bit of a fuss about it. We would like to believe that in the very near future there will be many more nurses echoing the sentiments of the nurse we quoted in Chapter 3: 'What's all the fuss about? What do people mean when they can't see how they'll fit in the time? I've had clinical supervision ever since I started nursing. To me it's as important as my annual leave: if I didn't have it, I'd be less effective at work, in fact I'd be ill. The same with clinical supervision: if I hadn't had it I'd have left nursing by now.'

References

Ahmad, W. (1992) *The Politics of Race and Health*. Bradford University: Race Relations Research Unit.

Ainsworth, M. (1982) Attachment: retrospect and prospect, in C.M. Parkes and J. Hinde (eds) *The Place of Attachment in Human Behavior*. New York: Basic Books.

Ainsworth, M., Blehar, M.C., Waters, E. and Wall, S. (1978) *Patterns of Attachment: Assessed in the Strange Situation and at Home*. Hillsdale, NJ: Erlbaum.

BAC (1993) *The Code of Ethics and Practice for Counsellors*. London: British Association for Counselling.

Bartholomew, K. and Perlman, D. (eds) (1994) *Attachment Processes in Adulthood*. London: Jessica Kingsley Publishers.

Belbin, R.M. (1981) *Management Teams: Why They Succeed or Fail*. Oxford: Heinemann.

Benner, P. (1984) *From Novice to Expert: Excellence and Power in Clinical Nursing Practice*. Reading, MA: Addison-Wesley.

Bent, A. (1992) The statutory basis to the role of the supervisor, in English National Board, *Preparation of Supervisors of Midwives*. London: English National Board.

Bentley, T. (1994) *Facilitation: Providing Opportunities for Learning*. London: McGraw-Hill.

Bion, W. (1967) *Second Thoughts: Selected Papers on Psychoanalysis*. Oxford: Heinemann Medical.

Blackburn, C. (1991) *Poverty and Health: Working with Families*. Buckingham: Open University Press.

Blackburn, C. (1992) *Improving Health and Welfare Work with Families in Poverty: A Handbook*. Buckingham: Open University Press.

Bond, M. (1986) *Stress and Self Awareness: A Guide for Nurses*. Oxford: Heinemann.

Bond, M. (1989) Managing emotional energy, in J. Mulligan (ed.) *The Personal Management Handbook*. London: Sphere.

Bond, M. (1991) Setting up groups: a practical guide, *Nursing Standard*, 21 August, 5(48): 47–51.

Bond, M. and Holland, S. (1992) *Communication in Partnership in Nutrifax*. London: Dairy Council and Community Practitioners and Health Visitors Association.

Boore, J. (1978) *Prescriptions for Recovery*. London: Royal College of Nursing.

Booth, K. and Faulkner, A. (1986) Problems encountered in setting up support groups in nursing, *Nursing Today*, 6: 244–51.

Boud, D. and Kilty, J. (1983) *Self and Peer Assessment in Higher Education: A Workshop Leader's Manual.* Sydney: Tertiary Education Centre, University of New South Wales.

Boud, D., Keogh, R. and Walker, D. (1985) Promoting reflection in learning: a model, in D. Boud, R. Keogh and D. Walker (eds) *Reflection: Turning Experience into Learning.* London: Kogan Page.

Bowlby, J. (1971) *Attachment and Loss*, vol. 1: *Attachment.* London: Hogarth Press.

Bowlby, J. (1973) *Attachment and Loss*, vol. 2: *Separation: Anxiety and Anger.* London: Hogarth Press.

Bowlby, J. (1980) *Attachment and Loss*, vol. 3: *Loss, Sadness and Depression.* London: Hogarth Press.

Bowlby, J. (1988) *A Secure Base: Clinical Applications of Attachment Theory.* London: Routledge.

Bretherton, I. and. Waters, E. (eds) (1985) *Growing Points of Attachment Theory and Research* (Monographs of the Society for Research in Child Development) 50(1–2), Serial No. 209.

Brown, A. and Bourne, I. (1996) *The Social Work Supervisor.* Buckingham: Open University Press.

Burnard, P. (1988) Mentors: a supporting act, *Nursing Times*, 83(2): 14–20.

Burnard, P. and Morrison, P. (1988) Nurses' perceptions of their interpersonal skills: a descriptive study using 6-Category Intervention Analysis, *Nurse Education Today*, 8: 272–86.

Butterworth, T. (1992) Clinical supervision . . . as an emerging idea in nursing, in T. Butterworth and J. Faugier (eds) *Clinical Supervision and Mentorship in Nursing.* London: Chapman and Hall.

Butterworth, T. (1995) Introduction to clinical supervision, in Department of Health, *Clinical Supervision – Conference Proceedings.* London: National Health Service Management Executive.

Butterworth, T. (1996) Primary attempts at research-based evaluation of clinical supervision, *Nursing Times Research*, 1(2): 96–101.

Butterworth, T., Carson, J., White, E., Jeacock, J., Clements, A. and Bishop, V. (1997) *It is Good to Talk: Clinical Supervision and Mentorship. An evaluation study in England and Scotland.* Manchester: University of Manchester.

Butterworth, T. and Faugier, J. (eds) (1992) *Clinical Supervision and Mentorship in Nursing.* London: Chapman and Hall.

Buttigieg, M. (1995) Foreword to G. Swain *Clinical Supervision: The Principles and Process.* London: Community Practitioners and Health Visitors Association.

Buzan, T. (1974) *Use Your Head.* London: BBC.

Buzan, T. and Buzan, B. (1995) *The Mind Map Book*, 2nd edn. London: BBC Books.

Campbell, F., Cowley, S. and Buttigieg, M. (1995) *Weights and Measures.* London: Community Practitioners and Health Visitors Association.

Carper, B. (1978) Fundamental ways of knowing in nursing, *Advances in Nursing Science*, 11: 13–23.

Carson, J., Fagin, L. and Ritter, S.A. (eds) (1995) *Stress and Coping in Mental Health Nursing.* London: Chapman and Hall.

Casement, P. (1985) *On Learning from the Patient.* London: Routledge.

Chavasse, J. (1992) New dimensions of empowerment in nursing, *Journal of Advanced Nursing*, 17: 1–2.

Checkland, P. (1970) *Systems Thinking, Systems Practice.* Chichester: John Wiley and Sons.

Chevannes, M. (1991) Access to health care for Black people, *Health Visitor*, 64(1): 16–18.

Clulow, C. (1994) Balancing care and control: the supervisory relationship as a focus for promoting organisational health, in A. Obholzer and V.Z. Roberts (eds) *The Unconscious at Work.* London: Routledge.

Cockman, P., Evans, B. and Reynolds, P. (1992) *Client Centred Consulting*. London: McGraw-Hill.

Cooper, C. (1981) *The Stress Check: Coping with the Stressors of Life and Work*. Englewood Cliffs, NJ: Spectrum Books, Prentice-Hall.

Cowley, S. (1993) Skill mix: value for whom?, *Health Visitor*, 66(5): 166–8.

Dartington, A. (1994) Where angels fear to tread: idealism, despondency and inhibition of thought in hospital nursing, in A. Obholzer and V.Z. Roberts (eds) *The Unconscious at Work*. London: Routledge.

Davies, C. (1995) *Gender and the Professional Predicament in Nursing*. Buckingham: Open University Press.

Department of Health (1991a) *A Study of Inquiry Reports into Child Abuse*. London: HMSO.

Department of Health (1991b) *Working Together Under the Children Act*. London: HMSO.

Department of Health (1991c) *The Patient's Charter*. London: HMSO.

Department of Health (1991d) *Equal Opportunities for Women in the NHS (Opportunity 2000)*. London: National Health Service Management Executive.

Department of Health (1993a) *A Vision for the Future*. London: National Health Service Management Executive.

Department of Health (1993b) *Ethnic Minority Staff in the NHS: A Programme for Action*. London: National Health Service Management Executive.

Department of Health (1993c) *The Patient's Charter and Primary Health Care*. London: HMSO.

Department of Health (1993d) *A Vision for the Future*. London: National Health Service Management Executive.

Department of Health (1994) *Guideline to Developing a Marketing Action Plan: Coopers and Lybrand/HVA*. London: HMSO.

Department of Health (1995) *Making It Happen: Public Health – the Contribution, Role and Development of Nurses, Midwives and Health Visitors*. London: HMSO.

Department of Health (1996a) *Clinical Supervision – A Resource Pack for Practice Nurses*. London: National Health Service Management Executive.

Department of Health (1996b) *Primary Care: The Future*. London: National Health Service Management Executive.

Dickson, A. (1982) *A Woman in Your Own Right: Assertiveness and You*. London: Quartet.

Dimond, B. (1990) *Legal Issues in Nursing*. Hemel Hempstead: Prentice-Hall.

Dimond, B. (1997a) Clinical supervision: the legal aspects 1, *Journal of Nursing* (in press).

Dimond, B. (1997b) Clinical supervision: the legal aspects 2, *Journal of Nursing* (in press).

Egan, G. (1975) *The Skilled Helper: A Model for Systematic Helping and Interpersonal Relating*. Monterey, CA: Brooks/Cole.

Elliott, P.A. (1995) Clinical supervision: advanced nursing practice through celebrating success and cascading confidence. Unpublished MSc thesis, University of Central England.

ENB (English National Board) (1992) *Preparation of Supervisors of Midwives*. London: English National Board.

Faugier, J. (1992) The supervisory relationship, in T. Butterworth and J. Faugier (eds) *Clinical Supervision and Mentorship in Nursing*. London: Chapman and Hall.

Faugier, J. (1995) Introduction to clinical supervision, in Department of Health, *Clinical Supervision – Conference Proceedings*. November 1994. London: National Health Service Management Executive.

Ferguson, K. (1992) Position paper on in-patient psychiatric nursing. Department of Health (unpublished).

Fernando, S. (ed.) (1995) *Mental Health in a Multi-Ethnic Society.* London: Routledge.

Fineman, S. (1993a) Organisations as emotional arenas, in S. Fineman (ed.) *Emotions in Organisations.* London: Sage.

Fineman, S. (ed.) (1993b). *Emotions in Organisations.* London: Sage.

Fish, D., Twinn, S. and Purr, B. (1989) *How to Enable Learning through Professional Practice.* London: West London Press.

Fowler, J. (1996) The organisation of clinical supervision within the nursing profession: a review of the literature, *Journal of Advanced Nursing,* 23: 471–8.

Freud, S. (1915) 'The unconscious', S.E. 14: 166–204. London: Hogarth Press.

Goldberg, N. (1986) *Writing Down the Bones: Freeing the Writer Within.* Boston, MA: Shambala.

Goleman, D. (1996) *Emotional Intelligence.* London: Bloomsbury.

Gregory, J. (1989) Self and peer assessment. *Welling, Kent Nurse Training Resource Interest Group Newsletter* No. 1 (April).

Gregory, J. (1996) *The Psychosocial Education of Nurses.* Aldershot: Avebury.

Grossman, K., Grossman, K.E., Spangler, G., Suess, G. and Unzer, J. (1985) Maternal sensitivity and newborns' orientation responses as related to quality of attachment in northern Germany, in I. Bretherton and E. Waters (eds) *Growing Points of Attachment Theory and Research* (Monographs of the Society for Research in Child Development) 50(1–2), Serial No. 209.

Guggenbuhl Craig, A. (1971) *Power in the Helping Professions,* Dallas, TX: Spring Publications.

Hall, D. (1996) *Health for All Children,* (3rd edn) (The Hall Report) Oxford: Oxford University Press.

Halton, W. (1994) Some unconscious aspects of organisational life, in A. Obholzer and V.Z. Roberts (eds) *The Unconscious at Work.* London: Routledge.

Handy, C. (1990) *Inside Organisations.* Harmondsworth: Penguin.

Hart, E. and Bond, M. (1993) *Action Research for Health and Social Care: A Guide to Practice.* Buckingham: Open University Press.

Hawkins, P. and Shohet, R. (1989) *Supervision in the Helping Professions.* Milton Keynes: Open University Press.

Hayward, J. (1975) *Information: A Prescription against Pain.* London: Royal College of Nursing.

Hearn, J. (1993) Emotive subjects; organisational men, organisational masculinities and the (de)construction of 'emotions', in S. Fineman (ed.) *Emotions in Organisations.* London: Sage.

Heron, J. (1972) *The Concept of a Peer Learning Community.* Guildford: Human Potential Resource Group, University of Surrey.

Heron, J. (1981) *Assessment.* Guildford: Human Potential Resource Group, University of Surrey.

Heron, J. (1983) *Education of the Affect.* Guildford: Human Potential Resource Group, University of Surrey.

Heron, J. (1989) *The Facilitator's Handbook.* London: Kogan Page.

Heron, J. (1990) *Helping the Client.* London: Sage.

Hill, J. (1989) Supervision in the caring professions: a literature review, *Community Psychiatric Nursing Journal,* 9(5): 9–15.

Hingley, P., Cooper, C.L. and Harris, P. (1986) *Stress in Nurse Managers.* London: King's Fund.

Holland, S. (1987) *Stress in Nursing.* London: Distance Learning Centre, South Bank University.

Holland, S. (1991) *Accountability in Health Visiting.* London: Community Practitioners and Health Visitors Association.

Holland, S. (1994) Returning to practice, *Health Visitor,* 67(3): 82–3.

Holland, S. (1995) *Reassessing Practice*. London: Community Practitioners and Health Visitors Association.

Houston, G. (1990) *Supervision and Counselling*. London: Rochester Foundation.

HVA (Health Visitors Association) (1994) *Action for Health: Marketing, Skill Mix, Campaigning*. London: Health Visitors Association.

Jacobsen, B., Smith, A. and Whitehead, M. (eds) (1991) *The Nation's Health: A Strategy for the 1990s*. London: King's Fund Centre.

Jacques, D. (1991) *Learning in Groups* (2nd edn). London: Kogan Page.

James, N. (1993) Divisions of emotional labour: disclosure and cancer, in S. Fineman (ed.) *Emotions in Organisations*. London: Sage.

Jarvis, P. (1983) *Professional Education*. Beckenham: Croom Helm.

Johns, C. (1994) Guided reflection in A. Palmer *et al.* (eds) *Reflective Practice in Nursing*. Oxford: Blackwell Science.

Johnson, D.W. and Johnson, F.P. (1987) *Joining Together: Group Theory and Group Skills* (3rd edn). Englewood Cliffs, NJ: Prentice Hall.

Johnson, P. (1995) The community services view, in Department of Health, *Clinical Supervision – Conference Proceedings*. London: National Health Service Management Executive.

Kadushin, A. (1992) *Supervision in Social Work* (3rd edn). New York: Columbia University Press.

Kendall, S. (1991) 'An analysis of Health Visitor/Client interaction: the influence of the HV process on client participation'. Unpublished PhD thesis, Kings College, London.

King's Fund (1997) *London's Mental Health: The Report to the King's Fund Commission*. London, King's Fund Centre.

Kohner, N. (1994) *Clinical Supervision in Practice*. London: King's Fund Centre.

Kolb, D.A. (1984) *Experiential Learning: Experience as the Source of Learning and Development*. Englewood Cliffs, NJ: Prentice Hall.

Kolb, D.A. and Fry, R. (1975) Towards an applied theory of experiential learning, in C.L. Cooper (ed.) *Theories of Group Processes*. Chichester: John Wiley.

Kraemer, S. and Roberts, J. (eds) (1996) *The Politics of Attachment*. London: Free Association Books.

Kramer, M. (1974) *Reality Shock: Why Nurses Leave Nursing*. St Louis, MI: C.V. Mosby.

Lewin, K. (1951) *Field Theory in Social Science*. London: Harper.

Lewin, K. (1972) Need, force and valence in psychological fields, in E.P. Hollander and R.G. Hunt (eds) *Classic Contributions to Social Psychology*. London: Oxford University Press.

Lightfoot, J., Baldwin, S. and Wright, K. (1992) *Nursing by Numbers*. University of York, Social Policy Research Unit.

Main, M. (1994) 'A move to the level of representation in the study of attachment organisation: implications for psychoanalysis'. Annual Research Lecture to the British Psycho-Analytical Society, July 1994.

Main, M. and Goldwyn, R. (1985) 'Adult attachment classification and rating system'. Unpublished manuscript, University of California, Berkeley.

Maroda, K.J. (1991) *The Power of Countertransference*. Chichester: John Wiley.

Marris, P. (1996) The management of uncertainty, in S. Kraemer and J. Roberts (eds) *The Politics of Attachment*. London: Free Asscociation Books.

Mattinson, J. (1975) *The Reflection Process in Casework Supervision*. London, Institute of Marital Studies.

Menzies, I. (1959) A case study in the functioning of social systems as a defence against anxiety: a report on a study of the nursing service of a general hospital, *Human Relations*, 13: 95–121.

Menzies-Lyth, I. (1988) *Containing Anxiety in Institutions*. London: Free Association Books.

Miyake, K., Chen, S. and Campos, J. (1985) Infant temperament, mother's mode of interaction, and attachment in Japan: an interim report, in I. Bretherton and E. Waters (eds) *Growing Points of Attachment Theory and Research* (Monographs of the Society for Research in Child Development) 50(1–2), Serial No. 209.

Morton-Cooper, A. and Palmer, A. (1993) *Mentoring and Preceptorship: A Guide to Support Roles in Clinical Practice*. Oxford: Blackwell Scientific Publications.

Mosse, J. and Roberts, V.Z. (1994) Finding a voice: differentiation, representation and empowerment in organisations under threat, in A. Obholzer and V.Z. Roberts (eds) *The Unconscious at Work*. London: Routledge.

Norman, A. (1993) Vested interests, *Nursing Times*, 89(50): 25–6.

Norman, A. (1995) Summing up of plenary session, in Department of Health, *Clinical Supervision – Conference Proceedings*. London: National Health Service Management Executive.

Obholzer, A. and Roberts, V.Z. (eds) (1994) *The Unconscious at Work*. London: Routledge.

Palmer, A., Burns, S. and Bulman, S. (eds) (1994) *Reflective Practice in Nursing*. Oxford: Blackwell Science.

Parkes, C.M., Hinde, J. and Marris, P. (eds) (1991) *Attachment Across the Life Cycle*. London: Routledge.

Parkin, W. (1993) The public and the private: gender, sexuality and emotion, in S. Fineman (ed.) *Emotions in Organisations*. London: Sage.

Parkinson, J. (1992) Supervision versus control: can managers provide both managerial and professional supervision?, in C. Cloke and J. Naish (eds) *Key Issues in Child Protection for Health Visitors and Nurses*. Harlow: Longman.

Pearson, A. (1988) 'Therapeutic nursing'. Unpublished PhD thesis, Burford and Oxford Nursing Development Unit.

Pedler, M., Burgoyne, J. and Boydell, T. (1991) *The Learning Company*. London: McGraw-Hill.

Platt-Koch, L.M. (1986) Clinical supervision for psychiatric nurses, *Journal of Psycho-Social Nursing* (January), 26(1): 7–15.

Proctor, B. (1987) Supervision: a co-operative exercise in accountability, in M. Marken and M. Payne (eds) *Enabling and Ensuring*. Leicester: National Youth Bureau for Education in Youth and Community Work.

Putnam, L. and Mumby, D. (1993) Organisations, emotion and the myth of rationality, in S. Fineman (ed.) (1993) *Emotions in Organisations*. London: Sage.

Rafferty, A.M. (1993) *Leading Questions: A Discussion Paper on Issues of Nurse Leadership*. London: King's Fund Centre.

Randall, R. and Southgate, J. (1980) *Cooperative and Community Group Dynamics . . . Or Your Meetings Needn't Be So Appalling*. London: Barefoot Books.

Reason, P. (1988) *Human Inquiry in Action: Developments in New Paradigm Research*. London: Sage.

Reason, P. and Rowan, J. (1981) *Human Inquiry*. Chichester: Wiley.

Revans, R.W. (1982) *The Origins and Growth of Action Learning*. Bromley, Kent: Chartwell-Bratt.

Roberts, V.Z. (1994) Till death us do part: caring and uncaring in work with the elderly, in A. Obholzer and V.Z. Roberts (eds) *The Unconscious at Work*. London: Routledge.

Robertson, J. and Robertson, J. (1989) *Separation and the Very Young*. London: Free Association Books.

Robinson, K. (1992) The nursing workforce: aspects of inequality, in J. Robinson, A. Gray and R. Elkan (eds) *Policy Issues in Nursing*. Buckingham: Open University Press.

Sagi, A., Lamb, E., Lewkowicz, S., Shoham, R., Dvir, R. and Estes, D. (1985) Security of infant, mother, father and metapelet attachments among kibbutz reared Israeli children, in I. Bretherton and E. Waters (eds) *Growing Points of Attachment Theory and*

Research (Monographs of the Society for Research in Child Development) 50(1–2), Serial No. 209.

Salvage, J. (1985) *The Politics of Nursing*. Oxford: Heinemann.

Salvage, J. (1992) The new nursing: empowering patients or empowering nurses?, in J. Robinson, A. Gray and R. Elkan (eds) *Policy Issues in Nursing*. Buckingham: Open University Press.

Schön, D. (1983) *The Reflective Practitioner*. New York: Basic Books.

Schön, D. (1987) *Educating the Reflective Practitioner*. San Francisco: Jossey-Bass.

Searles, H.F. (1955) The informational value of the supervisor's emotional experience, in *Collected Papers on Schizophrenia and Related Subjects*. London: Hogarth Press, 1965.

Skelton, R. (1994) Nursing and empowerment: concepts and strategies, *Journal of Advanced Nursing*, 19: 415–23.

Smith, P. (1992) *The Emotional Labour of Nursing*. London: Macmillan.

Sperling, M. and Berman, W. (1994) *Attachment in Adults*. New York: Guilford Press.

Sroufe, L.A., Egeland, B. and Kreutzer, T. (1990) The fate of early experience following developmental change: Longitudinal approaches to individual adaptation in childhood, *Child Development*, 61: 1363–73.

Stein, H. (1985) *The Psycho-Dynamics of Medical Practice: Unconscious Factors in Patient Care*. Los Angeles and London: University of California Press.

Stern, D. (1985) *The Interpersonal World of the Infant*. New York: Basic Books.

Stern, D. (1995) *The Motherhood Constellation: A Unified View of Parent–Infant Psychotherapy*. New York: Basic Books.

Swain, G. (1995) *Clinical Supervision: The Principles and Process*. London: Community Practitioners and Health Visitors Association.

Thomas, B. (1995) Clinical supervision in mental health nursing, in Department of Health, *Clinical Supervision – Conference Proceedings*. November 1994. London: National Health Service Management Executive.

Townsend, P. and Davidson, N. (1982) *Inequalites in Health: The Black Report and the Health Divide*. Harmondsworth: Penguin.

UKCC (1989) *Exercising Accountability – A Framework to Assist Nurses, Midwives and Health Visitors to Consider Ethical Aspects of Professional Practice* (3rd edn). London: United Kingdom Central Council for Nursing Midwifery and Health Visiting.

UKCC (1992a) *Code of Professional Conduct* (3rd edn). London: United Kingdom Central Council for Nursing Midwifery and Health Visiting.

UKCC (1992b) *The Scope of Professional Practice*. London: United Kingdom Central Council for Nursing Midwifery and Health Visiting.

UKCC (1993) *The Future of Professional Practice: The Council's Standards for Education and Practice Following Registration*. London: United Kingdom Central Council for Nursing Midwifery and Health Visiting.

UKCC (1996) *Position Statement on Clinical Supervision for Nursing and Health Visiting*. London: United Kingdom Central Council for Nursing Midwifery and Health Visiting.

Watkins, S. (1993) Working together for better health, *Health Visitor*, 66(12): 436–7.

White, E. (1990) *The Third Quinquennial National Community Psychiatric Nursing Survey*. Report. University of Manchester.

Whitehead, M. (1987) *The Health Divide*. London: Health Education Council.

Winnicott, D.W. (1991) *The Maturational Processes and the Facilitating Environment*. London: Hogarth.

Woodhouse, D. and Pengelly, P. (1991) *Anxiety and the Dynamics of Collaboration*. Newcastle: Aberdeen University Press.

Woods, D. (1992) The therapeutic use of self in clinical supervision, in T. Butterworth and J. Faugier (eds) *Clinical Supervision and Mentorship in Nursing*. London: Chapman and Hall.

Wynne, T. (1994) The burden facing women carers today, *Health Visitor*, 67(7): 241–2.

Index

Feedback about this book

Please post your answers to the following questions to:

Meg Bond and Stevie Holland
GO education – the Group and Open Education Consultancy
7 Cheverton Road
London
N19 3BB

1 What do you find most helpful about this book?

2 What do you find least helpful?

3 Any suggestions about further editions of this book or about further books?

4 What is your area of work?

5 Can we quote you in further editions of the book (a 'no' will be absolutely respected)?

Your replies will help us in planning further editions of the book and in designing our clinical supervision training courses.